T0182818

Nursing Practice in
Multiple Sclerosis

June Halper, MSN, APN-C, MSCN, FAAN, is a certified adult nurse practitioner who has specialized in multiple sclerosis (MS) since 1978. She was a founder of the MS Center in Teaneck, New Jersey, and was the executive director from its founding in 1985 through 2008. Ms. Halper is currently the CEO of the Consortium of Multiple Sclerosis Centers (CMSC) and the executive director of the International Organization of MS Nurses.

Ms. Halper has published and lectured extensively on multiple sclerosis and its ramifications. Her numerous publications include *Comprehensive Nursing Care in Multiple Sclerosis* and *Advanced Concepts in Nursing Care in Multiple Sclerosis*, and she was a coeditor of *Staying Well With Multiple Sclerosis: A Self-Care Guide* and *Nursing Practices in Multiple Sclerosis: A Core Curriculum.* She is a member of the American Academy of Nurse Practitioners, the founding director of the International Organization of MS Nurses (IOMSN), and the recipient of the IOMSN's first June Halper Award for Excellence in Nursing in Multiple Sclerosis. Ms. Halper continues to be involved in clinical care as a nurse practitioner at the MS Center of the New Jersey Medical School, Rutgers University, Newark, New Jersey, and at the Bergen Volunteer Medical Initiative in Hackensack, New Jersey. She is dedicated to the fight against MS through educating the next generation of health care professionals, as well as expanding research to promote best practices in the comprehensive management of the disease.

Colleen Harris, MN, NP, MSCN, is a nurse coordinator/nurse practitioner at the University of Calgary Multiple Sclerosis (MS) Clinic, where she has been involved in multidisciplinary care for much of her nursing career. She holds an adjunct assistant professor appointment with the faculty of nursing at the University of Calgary, where she is actively involved in both undergraduate and graduate nursing education. In addition to publishing numerous articles on MS and chronic illness, she has authored chapters in both *Comprehensive Nursing Care in Multiple Sclerosis* and *Advanced Concepts in Nursing Care in Multiple Sclerosis.*

Her interests specific to MS include intrathecal baclofen therapy, pain management, health outcomes research, and the development of multidisciplinary collaborative models of care.

Ms. Harris, along with several of her MS nursing colleagues from North America, Europe, and Australia, was involved in the creation of the International Organization of MS Nurses (IOMSN) and is one of the past presidents of the organization. She has been active in committee and project work with the Consortium of Multiple Sclerosis Centers (CMSC) for 25 years and was president of the organization from 2007 to 2009. She is the chair of the education committee of IOMSN, and under her leadership, the IOMSN has developed and conducted a wide variety of live, web-based, and enduring educational programs for nursing professionals.

Nursing Practice in Multiple Sclerosis

A Core Curriculum
Fourth Edition

June Halper, MSN, APN-C, MSCN, FAAN

Colleen Harris, MN, NP, MSCN

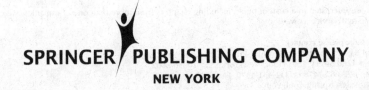

SPRINGER PUBLISHING COMPANY

NEW YORK

Copyright © 2017 Springer Publishing Company, LLC

All rights reserved.

No part of this publication may be reproduced, stored in a retrieval system, or transmitted in any form or by any means, electronic, mechanical, photocopying, recording, or otherwise, without the prior permission of Springer Publishing Company, LLC, or authorization through payment of the appropriate fees to the Copyright Clearance Center, Inc., 222 Rosewood Drive, Danvers, MA 01923, 978-750-8400, fax 978-646-8600, info@copyright.com or on the Web at www.copyright.com.

Springer Publishing Company, LLC
11 West 42nd Street
New York, NY 10036
www.springerpub.com

Acquisitions Editor: Margaret Zuccarini
Senior Managing Editor: Kris Parrish
Compositor: S4Carlisle Publishing Services

ISBN: 978-0-8261-3147-8
E-book ISBN: 978-0-8261-3148-5

16 17 18 19 20 / 5 4 3 2 1

The author and the publisher of this Work have made every effort to use sources believed to be reliable to provide information that is accurate and compatible with the standards generally accepted at the time of publication. Because medical science is continually advancing, our knowledge base continues to expand. Therefore, as new information becomes available, changes in procedures become necessary. We recommend that the reader always consult current research and specific institutional policies before performing any clinical procedure. The author and publisher shall not be liable for any special, consequential, or exemplary damages resulting, in whole or in part, from the readers' use of, or reliance on, the information contained in this book. The publisher has no responsibility for the persistence or accuracy of URLs for external or third-party Internet websites referred to in this publication and does not guarantee that any content on such websites is, or will remain, accurate or appropriate.

Library of Congress Cataloging-in-Publication Data

Names: Halper, June, author. | Harris, Colleen, author.
Title: Nursing practice in multiple sclerosis : a core curriculum / June
    Halper, Colleen Harris.
Description: Fourth edition. | New York : Springer Publishing Company, [2017]
    | Includes bibliographical references and index.
Identifiers: LCCN 2016021781| ISBN 9780826131478 | ISBN 9780826131485 (e-book)
Subjects: | MESH: Multiple Sclerosis--nursing
Classification: LCC RC377 | NLM WY 160.5 | DDC 616.8/340231--dc23 LC record available at
https://lccn.loc.gov/2016021781

Special discounts on bulk quantities of our books are available to corporations, professional associations, pharmaceutical companies, health care organizations, and other qualifying groups.

If you are interested in a custom book, including chapters from more than one of our titles, we can provide that service as well.

For details, please contact:
Special Sales Department, Springer Publishing Company, LLC
11 West 42nd Street, 15th Floor, New York, NY 10036-8002
Phone: 877-687-7476 or 212-431-4370; Fax: 212-941-7842
E-mail: sales@springerpub.com

Printed in the United States of America by Gasch Printing.

Contents

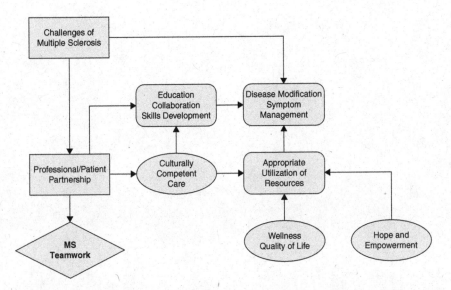

Multiple sclerosis (MS) nursing requires new and innovative strategies and structure to meet the complex needs of MS nursing professionals, who range from licensed practical nurses (LPNs) and RNs to advanced practice nurses (nurse practitioners and clinical nurse specialists). The content of this book focuses on the knowledge that MS nursing professionals need to support their professional growth and development. This nursing specialty has evolved from an underrecognized cadre of historic figures in multiple sclerosis to a broad spectrum of nursing professionals who practice throughout the world.

Linda Morgante set the stage for us by investigating the concept of hope in MS, a disease with enormous implications for patients and families as well as the health care community. We have adopted the model of care shown in the preceding figure into this work, as well as all of our other publications. This model incorporates the domains of MS nursing—clinical care, education, research, and advocacy—into an algorithm that has the leitmotif of hope throughout all nursing activities.

June Halper and Colleen Harris

Acknowledgments

We would like to thank Jenet Mesina for her invaluable assistance in the preparation of this book for publication.

I

Background Information for Nursing Practice in Multiple Sclerosis

1

The History of Multiple Sclerosis Care

OBJECTIVES

Upon completion of this chapter, the learner will be able to:

- *Identify the evolution of knowledge that has impacted the care of people with multiple sclerosis (MS)*
- *Discuss turning points in the definition and diagnosis of MS*

- Multiple sclerosis (MS) is a common neurologic disorder of young adults. It affects people in the prime of their lives with unpredictability, variability, and uncertainty. It is thought to affect more than 2.1 million people worldwide.

Age range is 10 to 65 years, with the highest incidence between 30 and 50 years, although it can present in children and older adults. It affects women close to three times as often as men.

- In recent decades, the *reputation* of MS as a disease with unrelenting progression has been modified owing to the impact of disease-modifying therapies for relapsing and worsening relapsing forms of the disease.

3

- Historically, it was known as a *peculiar disease state* (Robert Carswell), a *gray degeneration of the cord* (Jean Cruveilhier), and *insular sclerosis* (William Moxon and William Osler).

- *Disseminated sclerosis* was a term used in the early part of the 20th century.

- The name *multiple sclerosis* is a derivation from the German *multiple sklerose.*

- Early cases were as follows:

    A. Saint Lidwina van Schiedam

    B. Halla, the drummer Bock, and William Brown, a Hudson Bay official

    C. Sir Augustus d'Este

    D. Heinrich Heine

    E. Margaret Gatty

    F. W. N. P. Barbellion

- An early monograph on MS was written by Charles Prosper Ollivier.

- Other writings on MS were by Robert Carswell, Jean Cruveilhier, Marshall Hall, and others. These included anatomic depictions of autopsy findings, and the description included a clinical history.

- In 1868, Jean-Martin Charcot framed the disease and thoroughly described the clinical and pathologic features of MS. He added his own observations to those of Carswell, Cruveilhier, and the German physician von Frerichs, calling the disease *le sclerose en plaques,* or "scarring in patches."

- In 1873, Dr. Moxon, in England, characterized the disease based on observations.

- In 1878, Dr. Ranvier discovered myelin.

- For more than 100 years, physicians were frustrated trying to identify the cause of MS. Theories of causation ranged from infection to genetics, vascular problems, and immunologic deficits.

- In 1916, Dr. Dawson, at the University of Edinburgh in Scotland, used a microscope to describe inflammation around the blood vessels and the damage to the myelin with a clarity and thoroughness that has never been surpassed. Little was known then about the brain's function, so the meaning of these changes was only a guess.

- In 1919, abnormalities in cerebrospinal fluid were observed. The significance was unknown.

- In 1925, the first electrical recording of nerve transmission was made by Lord Edgar Douglas Adrian. The science of electrophysiology established techniques needed to study nerves.

- In 1928, myelin was studied under a microscope; oligodendrocytes (cells that produce myelin) were discovered.

▪ In 1935, Dr. Rivers, at the Rockefeller Institute in New York, reproduced the autoimmune response classically seen in MS. An animal model for MS was developed, called *experimental allergic encephalomyelitis.*

▪ Dietary modification was studied with no conclusive evidence of benefit.

▪ Alternative or complementary therapies emerged as frequently used supplements or substitutes for conventional treatments.

▪ In 1946, Sylvia Lawry founded the National Multiple Sclerosis Society (NMSS) in New York City, which has expanded into a worldwide network of MS societies. Services and programs include a wide range of patient and family services, basic and psychosocial research, and MS education. NMSS and the Canadian MS Society cover North America with a wide range of programs and services. The International Federation of Multiple Sclerosis Societies has member organizations worldwide.

▪ Dr. Kabat, at Columbia University, received the first NMSS grant to study MS.

▪ Dr. Salk received an NMSS grant to study the immunology of MS.

▪ In 1950, NMSS helped to establish a new division of the National Institutes of Health, called the National Institute for Neurologic Disorders and Stroke.

▪ In 1967, Ms. Lawry founded the International Federation of MS Societies, now the Multiple Sclerosis International Federation, which links MS societies around the world.

▪ In 1969, the first successful clinical trial in the treatment of MS was studied.

A. It was placebo controlled.

B. New rating scales and diagnostic standards were used.

C. Patients were given adrenocorticotropic hormone (ACTH) or a placebo.

▪ In the 1970s, research produced useful results.

A. Scientists studying experimental allergic encephalomyelitis (EAE), an animal model thought to resemble MS, suspected that myelin protein fragments might prevent the disease.

B. A mixture of the fragments was used to treat animals and then humans with MS (copolymer 1).

C. Steroids became more widely used to suppress the immune response.

D. In 1978, computed tomography (CT) scanning was first used for MS patients.

E. First experiments with interferons demonstrated their immunomodulating effects. Dr. Larry Jacobs, in Buffalo, was an early leader in researching this innovative treatment.

F. In the 1980s, Dr. Howard Weiner, in Boston, studied cyclophosphamide in MS. Although never given U.S. Food and Drug Administration

(FDA) approval as an immunosuppressant in MS, it is still widely used in clinical settings.

G. During the 1970s, the emergence of new treatments and diagnostic techniques led to the proliferation of MS treatment centers throughout North America and the beginnings of the team approach to MS care.

■ The 1980s saw the beginnings of major clinical trials in MS using immunomodulators, such as interferons and glatiramer acetate (copolymer 1).

■ Dr. Young performed the first MRI on a patient with MS.

■ In 1984, it became apparent that MRI can visualize MS attacks in the brain, including many that did not manifest symptoms.

■ In 1986, the Consortium of Multiple Sclerosis Centers (CMSC) was founded. The CMSC is the largest organization of MS health professionals in the world. It holds annual and regional meetings, consensus conferences, and training programs for MS professionals. It has a journal, *International Journal of MS Care*, that is both in print and online. The CMSC Foundation funds scholarships and fellowships in MS training; the CMSC North American Research Committee on Multiple Sclerosis project (NARCOMS) has a large patient-driven database to increase understanding of MS and its ramifications. NARCOMS, a clinician-driven registry, was established in 2014.

INTERNATIONAL MS PROFESSIONAL ORGANIZATIONS

In 1984, the European Committee for Treatment and Research in Multiple Sclerosis (ECTRIMS) was founded and held annual scientific meetings in Europe. The Americas Committee for Treatment and Research in Multiple Sclerosis (ACTRIMS), the North American counterpart, was established in 1995, followed by LACTRIMS, a Latin American organization representing Central and South America.

In 1991, Rehabilitation in Multiple Sclerosis (RIMS), a European network, was created.

Subsequently, PCTRIMS, covering the Pacific Rim countries, and BCTRIMS, in Brazil, represented care and research in their respective areas of the world. In 2014 and 2015, MENACTRIMS, representing the Middle East and northern Africa, held its first meetings.

■ In 1993, the FDA approved Betaseron (interferon beta-1b) for relapsing–remitting MS (R–R MS) (Bayer Healthcare, Whippany, NJ).

■ In 1996, Avonex (interferon beta-1a IM) was approved for R–R MS (Biogen, Cambridge, MA).

■ In 1996, Copaxone (glatiramer acetate) was approved for R–R MS (Teva Neuroscience, Kansas City, MO).

■ In 1997, the International Organization of Multiple Sclerosis Nurses (IOMSN) was founded (www.iomsn.org). The following are the goals and strategies of the IOMSN:

A. Facilitate the development of a specialized branch of nursing in MS

   1. Develop and maintain a mechanism by which members can share information on practice positions and resources

   2. Establish the IOMSN as a forum for discussion and collaboration on issues that concern MS nurses

   3. Serve as a resource for external organizations related to MS practice issues

   4. Promote the acknowledgment of the contribution of IOMSN as the preeminent organization of MS nurses

   5. Participate with other nursing organizations involved in MS care or related fields

   6. Share information on research activities among members

B. Establish standards of nursing care in MS

   1. Develop minimal standards of nursing practice in MS

   2. Facilitate the development of a core curriculum for MS nursing to disseminate this information

   3. Identify specific domains of MS nursing and define basic roles and responsibilities in each domain

C. Support MS nursing research, basic research, and clinical trials

   1. Encourage research activities that contribute to the development of a sound theoretical basis for MS practice

   2. Recommend research topics for educational sessions at IOMSN meetings for dissemination of evidence-based information

   3. Develop and implement nursing research

   4. Disseminate MS nursing research findings through publications and educational activities

D. Educate the health care community about MS

   1. Promote communication among the IOMSN membership via the newsletter, the Web site, and other avenues

   2. Facilitate internal and external communication about MS care and research

■ MS nursing organizations exist in Sweden, Italy, Finland, Australia, and The Netherlands.

- Multiple Sclerosis International Credentialing Board was founded in 2001.

    A. The Multiple Sclerosis International Credentialing Board is responsible for the development and administration of the certification examination in MS nursing.

    B. The IOMSN endorses the concept of voluntary certification by examination for all nursing professionals providing care in MS. Those who work or have worked in this specialty and meet eligibility requirements may take this examination. Certification focuses specifically on the individual and is an indication of knowledge and skills and MS practice. MS nursing certification provides formal recognition of a level of knowledge in the field and promotes the delivery of safe and effective practice in the domains of clinical practice (disease course and classifications, epidemiology, and distribution), advocacy (ethical practice, negotiating the health care system, empowerment, knowledge of community resources, patient rights, and consultation expertise), education (principles of teaching and learning, health promotion and change theory, special populations, and professional development), and research (evidence-based practice, protection of human subjects, and research terminology and process).

    C. All candidates must be licensed nursing professionals with at least 2 years' experience in MS. Candidates must also agree to adhere to the IOMSN Code of Ethics.

    D. The basic content of the examination covers the following:
    1. Basic concepts of MS (disease course classification, pathophysiology of MS, and diagnostic process)
    2. Pharmacologic and nonpharmacologic treatment
    3. Symptom management
    4. Psychosocial intervention
    5. Research and education initiatives
    6. Patient advocacy

- In 2000, mitoxantrone (Novantrone) was approved for worsening forms of relapsing MS.
- In 2003, the CMSC issued its recommendations for MS Care (see Appendix B).
- In 2003, the United Kingdom Multiple Sclerosis Specialist Nurse Association (ukmssna@mstrust.org.uk) was founded.

    A. The goals and mission are similar to those of IOMSN.

    B. The United Kingdom Multiple Sclerosis Specialist Nurse Association (UKMSSNA) has representation on the IOMSN board.

■ The Multiple Sclerosis Certified Specialist (MSCS) examination was developed by the Clinical Care Committee of the CMSC in 2003 to 2004. The first examination was offered in 2004 for MS specialists (not registered nurses).

A. Content of the examination includes concepts of rehabilitation, emotional issues, long-term care, and the above topics.

B. Certification will validate expertise by examination of the multidisciplinary, interdisciplinary MS team.

A FLOW OF DISEASE MODIFYING THERAPIES FOR RELAPSING MS

In 2002, Rebif (interferon-β 1-a SQ) was approved for R–R MS (EMD Serono, Rockland, MA).

In 2004, Tysabri (natalizumab) was approved for relapsing forms of MS. It was withdrawn from the market in early 2005 because of safety concerns (discussed further in this book). It was re–released in 2006 with monitoring procedures in place.

In 2010, the first oral symptomatic medication, Ampryra (dalfampridine), was approved by the FDA to improve walking in MS.

In 2010, Gilenya (fingolimod), an oral disease-modifying therapy, entered the market for relapsing forms of MS (Novartis Pharmaceuticals, East Hanover, NJ).

In 2012, another oral medication, Aubagio (teriflunomide) was approved for relapsing MS (Genzyme Corporation, Boston, MA).

In 2014, Tecfidera (dimethyl fumarate), another oral therapy, reached the market for relapsing MS (Biogen, Cambridge, MA).

In 2014, Plegridy, a pegylated formation of Avonex, was approved by the FDA as a subcutaneous injection to be delivered every 2 weeks (Biogen, Cambridge, MA).

In late 2014, Lemtrada (alemtuzumab), an infusible therapy, was approved for worsening MS (Genzyme Corporation, Boston, MA). Special safety procedures and a Risk Evaluation and Mitigation Strategies (REMS) program are required for its administration and monitoring.

In mid-2015, Glatopa, a generic formulation of glatiramer acetetate, was approved by the FDA (Novartis Pharmaceuticals, East Hanover, NJ).

In mid-2016 Zinbryta™ (daclizumab) was approved for relapsing MS (Biogen, Cambrdige, MA; Abbvie, North Chicago, IL).

■ In 2015, in recognition of disorders resembling MS but distinct from this condition, a certification examination for rare neuroimmunologic disorders was developed. The first examination was offered in July 2015 for the multidisciplinary team with the designation CRND that examined the characteristics of MS mimickers such as the neuromyelitis optica (NMO) spectrum.

RESOURCES

Cutter, G., Yadavalli, R., Marrie, R. A., Tyry, T., Campagnolo, D., Bullock, B., & Vollmer, T. (2007). Changes in the sex ratio over time in multiple sclerosis. *Neurology, 68*(Suppl.), 162.

Halper, J. (2007). The nature of multiple sclerosis. In J. Halper (Ed.), Advanced concepts in multiple sclerosis nursing care (pp. 1–26). New York, NY: Demos Medical.

Halper, J., & Holland, N. J. (2011). An overview of multiple sclerosis. In J. Halper & N. J. Holland (Eds.), *Comprehensive nursing care in multiple sclerosis* (pp. 1–27). New York, NY: Springer Publishing.

Harris, C. J., & Halper, J. (2008). *Multiple sclerosis: Best practices in nursing care.* New York, NY: Bioscience Communications.

Murray, T. J. (2005). *Multiple sclerosis: The history of a disease.* New York, NY: Demos Medical.

Noonan, C. W., Williamson, D. M., Henry, J. P., Indian, R., Lynch, S. G., Neuberger, J. S., . . . Marrie, R. A. (2010). The prevalence of multiple sclerosis in 3 US communities. *Preventing Chronic Disease, 7,* A12.

Pittock, S. J. (2009). Clinical features and natural history of multiple sclerosis: The nature of the beast. In C. F. Lucchinetti & R. Hohlfeld (Eds.), *Multiple sclerosis 3* (pp. 1–18). Philadelphia, PA: Saunders.

Polman, C. H., Reingold, S. C., Banwell, B., Clanet, M., Cohen, J. A., Filippi, M., . . . Wolinsky, J. S. (2011). Diagnostic criteria for multiple sclerosis: 2010 revisions to the McDonald Criteria. *Annals of Neurology, 69,* 292–302.

Polman, C. H., Reingold, S. C., Edan, G., Filippi, M., Hartung, H. P., Kappos, L., . . . Wolinsky, J. S. (2005). Diagnostic criteria for multiple sclerosis: 2005 revisions to the "McDonald Criteria." *Annals of Neurology, 58,* 840–846.

Polman, C. H., Thompson, A. J., Murray, T. J., & McDonald, W. I. (2001). *Multiple sclerosis: The guide to treatment and management* (5th ed.). New York, NY: Demos Medical.

Warren, S., Turpin, K., Janzen, W., Warren, K., & Marrie, R. A. (2010, October 15). *Variance in health-related quality of life explained by socio-demographic and MS-related factors: Data from the North American Research Committee in Multiple Sclerosis.* Paper presented at the ECTRIMS 2010 Annual Meeting, Goteborg, Sweden.

2

Domains of Multiple Sclerosis Nursing Practice

OBJECTIVES

Upon completion of this chapter, the learner will be able to:

- List the four domains of multiple sclerosis (MS) nursing
- Describe nursing activities related to the core of care
- Cite professional responsibilities required to sustain the MS nursing role

- Nursing domains are considered the full range of nursing practice that may be called into use to serve the patient with multiple sclerosis (MS) and his or her family.
- MS practice domains are broad areas of accountability.
- Broad areas of practice include the full range of knowledge, skills, and tasks of MS nursing responsibility.
  A. It is important to recognize the unique nature of MS and its chronic and dynamic nature.
  B. Planning and implementing care requires flexibility, cultural sensitivity, and an ability to relate closely to the patient and family.

■ The domains of MS nursing include the following:
   A. Clinical practice
   B. Advocacy
   C. Education
   D. Research

■ The universal tasks of MS nursing are as follows:
   A. Establishment of a therapeutic partnership
   B. Performance of a comprehensive assessment
   C. Formulation of a collaborative treatment plan
   D. Initiation, facilitation, and maintenance of a treatment regimen
   E. Evaluation of a treatment plan

■ Domain: Clinical practice—knowledge
   A. Pathophysiology of disease
      1. Immune dysfunction
      2. Nerve conduction
   B. Definition, course, and classification
   C. Epidemiology and distribution
   D. Symptomatology
   E. Diagnosis of MS
      1. Presenting symptoms
      2. Prognostic indicators
      3. Diagnostic tests

■ Clinical practice—knowledge and skills
   A. Relapse management
   B. Disease-modifying agents
   C. Symptoms and symptom management
   D. Psychosocial issues

■ Domain: Advocacy
   A. Advocacy tasks
      1. Negotiate for the patient and family in the health care system
      2. Advocate self-care strategies
      3. Serve as a consultant

        4. Increase awareness of MS in the community

        5. Protect patient rights

        6. Examine practice outcomes

    B. Advocacy requires knowledge and skills

        1. Patient rights

        2. Ethical practice

        3. Negotiating the health care system

        4. Empowerment

        5. Public speaking

        6. Local and national health policy

        7. Disease expertise

■ Domain: Education

    A. Patient education

        1. Knowledge of MS

        2. Nursing process and theory

        3. Principles of teaching and learning

    B. Professional development

        1. Role model

        2. Mentor

        3. Preceptor

        4. Public speaker

        5. Support group leader

        6. Writer

        7. Membership in professional organizations

■ Domain: Research

    A. Knowledge of research terminology and process

    B. Protection of human subjects

    C. Evidence-based practice

    D. Research tasks and skills

        1. Proper sample collection

        2. Preparation and documentation

        3. Communication skills

        4. Research design, ethical principles

        5. Drive to increase nursing body of knowledge

MS NURSING PERFORMANCE ACTIVITIES

Assessment

■ The MS nurse collects and assesses patient health data.

MEASUREMENT CRITERIA

■ Data collection involves the patient, family, and other health care providers as appropriate.

■ The priority of data collection activities is determined by the patient's
immediate condition or needs.

■ Patient data are collected and assessed using appropriate assessment
techniques and instruments such as physical assessment, documentation
review, and interviews as appropriate to licensure and level of practice.

■ Relevant data are documented in a retrievable form.

■ The data collection process is systematic and ongoing. It is based on a
working knowledge of the effects of MS and the manifestation of those
effects.

Nursing Diagnosis

■ The MS nurse analyzes patient health data and determines nursing
diagnoses.

MEASUREMENT CRITERIA

■ Diagnoses are derived from the assessment data. Diagnoses address
all issues that are pertinent to the patient's health and success in the
family, the workplace, and the community. Diagnoses may include the
identification of actual or potential responses or illness with pertinent
etiologies or risk factors, with regard to the following:

A. Alterations in physical status, including complex assessment of organ systems, bowel and bladder functional assessment, respiratory
deficits, and muscle and sensory loss or alteration

B. Status of self-care activities, rehabilitation potential, functional level
ability, and potential functional ability

C. Emotional stress or crisis components of disability, pain, self-concept,
and individual and family development states

D. Alterations in thinking, perception, communication, and decision
making

E. Adaptation to and coping with alterations due to disability, durable
medical equipment, home, and lifestyle changes

F. Educational assessment of patient, family, and other care providers

G. Age-related and cultural issues

■ Diagnoses are validated with the patient, family, significant other, and other health care providers, when possible and appropriate.

■ Diagnoses are documented in a manner that facilitates the determination of optimal health care, expected outcomes, and plan of care.

Outcome Identification

■ The MS nurse identifies expected outcomes individualized to the patient.

MEASUREMENT CRITERIA

■ Outcomes are derived from the diagnoses. Expected outcomes are based on scientific knowledge about the outcomes of MS.

■ Outcomes are mutually formulated with the patient, family, and other health care providers when possible and appropriate.

■ Outcomes focus on maintaining an optimal level of functioning and independence, promoting health and quality of life, and preventing complications throughout the life span.

■ Outcomes are culturally appropriate and realistic in relation to the patient's present and potential capabilities.

■ Outcomes are attainable in relation to resources available to the patient.

■ Outcomes include a time estimate for attainment.

■ Outcomes provide direction for continuity of care.

■ Outcomes are documented as measurable.

■ Outcomes are assessed and amended throughout the person's lifetime with MS.

Planning

■ The MS nurse develops a plan of care that prescribes interventions to attain expected outcomes.

MEASUREMENT CRITERIA

■ The plan is individualized to the patient in terms of age, cultural and ethnic background, level of education, and needs.

- The plan is developed collaboratively with the patient, family, and other team members.
- The plan is comprehensive and addresses current and potential problems, as well as the maintenance of health and wellness and the prevention of complications.
- The plan reflects current MS practice.
- The plan is evolving and can be adapted to address changes.
- The plan provides for continuity of care.
- Priorities for care are established.
- The plan is documented.

Implementation

- The MS nurse implements the interventions identified in the plan of care.

MEASUREMENT CRITERIA

- Interventions are consistent with the established plan of care.
- Interventions are implemented in a safe, timely, and appropriate manner.
- Interventions are reviewed and modified on the basis of patient progress or change in condition.
- Interventions are documented.
- Interventions are derived using a team approach.

Evaluation

- The MS nurse evaluates the patient's progress toward attainment of outcomes.

MEASUREMENT CRITERIA

- Evaluation is systematic, ongoing, and criterion based.
- The patient, family, and other MS team members are involved as appropriate.
- Ongoing assessment data are used to revise the plan of care, interventions, and accomplishment of appropriate outcomes.
- Revisions are documented and communicated to the patient, family, and other team members.

- The effectiveness of interventions is evaluated in relation to outcomes.
- The patient's responses to interventions are documented.

PROFESSIONAL PERFORMANCE

Quality of Care

- The MS nurse systematically evaluates the quality of effectiveness of MS nursing practice.

MEASUREMENT CRITERIA

- The nurse participates in quality of care/performance improvement activities such as the following:
  A. Identifying aspects of care that are important for quality monitoring
  B. Identifying indicators used to monitor quality and effectiveness of nursing care
  C. Collecting data
  D. Analyzing quality data
  E. Formulating recommendations to improve nursing practice or patient outcomes
  F. Participating in interdisciplinary MS care
  G. Implementing activities to enhance the quality of MS nursing practice
  H. Developing policies and procedures to improve quality of care.

- The nurse uses the results of quality of care/performance improvement activities to initiate change in practice.
- The nurse uses the results of activities to initiate change throughout the health care system when appropriate.

Performance Appraisal

- The MS nurse evaluates nursing practice in relation to professional standards and relevant statutes and regulations.
- The nurse engages in performance appraisal on a regular basis.
- The nurse seeks constructive feedback.
- The nurse takes action to achieve goals identified in performance appraisals.
- The nurse participates in peer review.
- The nurse's practice reflects knowledge of current professional standards, laws, and regulations.

Education

■ The MS nurse acquires and maintains current knowledge and competency in nursing practice.

MEASUREMENT CRITERIA

■ The nurse participates in ongoing educational activities.

■ The nurse seeks experiences that reflect current clinical practice to maintain current clinical skills and competency.

■ The nurse acquires knowledge and skills appropriate to the specialty and practice setting.

Collegiality

■ The MS nurse interacts with peers and other colleagues and contributes to their professional development.

MEASUREMENT CRITERIA

■ The nurse shares knowledge and skills with colleagues.

■ The nurse provides colleagues with constructive feedback.

■ The nurse interacts with colleagues to enhance MS nursing practice.

■ The nurse facilitates the education of nursing and other health care students.

■ The nurse promotes a supportive, safe, and healthy work environment.

Ethics

■ The MS nurse's decision and actions on behalf of patients are determined in an ethical manner.

■ The nurse maintains patient privacy and confidentiality within legal and regulatory parameters.

■ The nurse acts as a patient advocate and assists the patient to develop skills to advocate for himself or herself.

■ The nurse delivers care in a nonjudgmental and nondiscriminatory manner and is sensitive to patient diversity, including age-related and cultural issues.

■ The nurse delivers care in a manner that preserves patient autonomy, dignity, and rights.

■ The nurse seeks available resources in formulating ethical decisions.

Collaboration

- The MS nurse collaborates with the patient and other health care providers in providing care.
- The nurse communicates with the patient, family, and other members of the health care team.
- The nurse collaborates to develop goals, plan of care, and decisions related to delivery of care.
- The nurse consults with other health care providers as needed.
- The nurse makes referrals to ensure continuity of care as needed.

Research

- The MS nurse integrates research findings into practice.
- The nurse uses evidence-based guidelines and research data in nursing practice.
- The nurse participates in research activities, as appropriate to the nurse's education and position. Such activities may include the following:
  - A. Identifying clinical problems suitable for nursing research
  - B. Participating in data collection
  - C. Participating in collaborative research activities
  - D. Disseminating research findings
  - E. Conducting research
  - F. Critiquing research for application to practice
  - G. Using research in the development of policies and procedures.

Resource Utilization

- The MS nurse considers factors related to safety, effectiveness, and cost in planning and delivering patient care.

MEASUREMENT CRITERIA

- The nurse evaluates factors related to safety, effectiveness, availability, and cost to determine practice options that would result in the same patient outcome.
- The nurse assists the patient and family in identifying and securing appropriate and available services for health-related needs.
- The nurse assigns or delegates tasks as defined by the state nurse practice acts and according to the knowledge and skills competency of the designated caregiver.

- If the nurse assigns or delegates tasks, it is based on the needs and condition of the patient, the potential for harm, the stability of the patient's condition, the complexity of the task, and the predictability of the outcome.
- The nurse assists the patient and the family to become informed consumers about the costs, risks, and benefits of treatment and care.

THE MULTIPLE SCLEROSIS SPECIALIST NURSE ASSOCIATION

Competencies for MS Specialist Nurses

The role of the MS specialist nurse, as defined by the United Kingdom organization representing MS specialist nurses (2003), is to "empower those affected by MS by providing information, support and advice about the condition from time of diagnosis and through the disease spectrum. The MS specialist nurse is pivotal in providing a greater understanding of the condition, and by adopting a holistic, collaborative and coordinated approach to help those individuals, where possible, reach their goals of self-management. The role involves acting as a consultant, an educational resource for staff, and striving towards great awareness and knowledge of MS in the health and social arena."

- Levels of competency were defined as follows:
  A. Novice
  B. Competent
  C. Expert

- Timelines were for the following:
  A. Novice up to 9 months from starting
  B. Competent 9 months onward
  C. Expert depending on the ability of the individual and working environment

- Areas of competency consisted of the following:
  A. Clinical management of MS
     1. Diagnostic phase
     2. Minimal impairment phase
     3. Moderate disability phase
     4. Severe disability phase

  B. Knowledge of MS
     1. Etiology of the disease
     2. Classification of disease course

    3. Pathology of the disease

    4. Comprehensive management

       a. Relapses

       b. Symptoms

       c. Treatment options

       d. Complementary therapies

       e. Possible adverse events

    5. Outcome measurement

    6. Cognitive impact

C. Relationships with people with MS and their families

    1. Trust and self-management

    2. Advocacy

    3. User service development

    4. Telephone management relationships and time management

D. Personal planning and organization

    1. Time management

    2. Administration support

E. Working in different health and social environments

    1. Integration and development of services

    2. Community and primary care etiquette

F. Accountability

    1. Scope of practice

    2. Accountability for service demands

    3. Documentation

    4. Evidence-based practice

    5. Informed consent

G. Teaching and sharing knowledge

    1. Development of educational programs

    2. Teaching

    3. Use of evaluation tools

    4. Mentorship

    5. Teaching people with MS

H. Audit

    1. Using research

    2. Doing research

   3. Patient trials
   4. Audit
 I. Relationships with professionals
   1. Partnerships
   2. Influence and leadership
   3. Professional networking
   4. Relationships with industry
 J. Professional and personal development
   1. Reflective practice
   2. Developing knowledge

RESOURCES

American Association of Spinal Cord Injury Nurses. (2004). *American Association of Spinal Cord Injury Nurses standards of practice—Revised 2003–2004. SCI Nursing, 21*(4), 228–232.

American Nurses Association. (2003). *Code of ethics for nurses with interpretive statement.* Washington, DC: American Nurses Publishing.

Burgess, M. (2002). *Multiple sclerosis: Theory and practice for nurses.* London, UK: Whurr Publishers.

Costello, K., & Halper, J. (2010a). *Multiple sclerosis: Key issues in nursing management.* New York, NY: EME.

Costello, K., & Halper, J. (2010b). *Advanced practice nursing in multiple sclerosis: Advanced skills, advancing responsibilities.* New York, NY: EME.

Multiple Sclerosis Trust. (2001). *Multiple sclerosis information for health and social care professionals.* Letchworth, UK: Author.

United Kingdom Multiple Sclerosis Specialist Nurse Association and the Multiple Sclerosis Trust. (2003). *Competencies for MS specialist nurses.* Letchworth, UK: Author.

3

Change Theory and Its Application in Multiple Sclerosis Nursing

OBJECTIVES

Upon completion of this chapter, the learner will be able to:

- Discuss the conceptual framework of change theory
  - *The models that facilitate critical thinking in multiple sclerosis (MS) nursing*
  - *Specifics relevant to health care behaviors*
- Describe its application in MS nursing
  - *Facilitating patient adherence to complex protocols with individualized nursing interventions*

- It is important to recognize the levels of health behavior.
- Primary prevention, in which a person tries to maximize wellness and avoid illness.
- Secondary prevention, in which a person's behaviors are meant to forestall complications.
- Tertiary prevention, in which one tries to control disease progression, comorbidities, or complications.

■ There are a number of theoretical models that are constructs of beliefs and attitudes.

A. The Health Belief Model, which focuses on a person's beliefs as a motivator of health behavior and employs the concept of self-efficacy

B. The Theory of Reasoned Action, which attempts to explain attitudes and actions that a person undertakes

C. The Transtheoretical Model of Change, which involves increasing a person's awareness of the situation.

D. The Social Cognitive Model, which employs elements such as self-efficacy and empowerment.

■ During change, the person who is the change agent (multiple sclerosis [MS] nurse) interacts with the patient's system (values and beliefs) to influence change and adaptation.

■ Thus, the nurse as a change agent must be especially sensitive to feedback to determine how activities, ideas, and new programs are being accepted.

■ Change must be planned with respect for the environment, social and economic factors, ethnocultural concerns, and resources.

■ The role of change agent is a challenging opportunity for nursing. Power is derived either from relationships, cultural sensitivity, knowledge and expertise, or all of these factors.

■ One must consider the unique and highly personal values of each individual to initiate change.

■ Resistance to change can be minimized if the nurse keeps the interactions open and dynamic.

■ It is important to acknowledge the following factors that the patient and nurse must face when dealing with the dynamic nature of MS:

A. Adapting to new lifestyles

B. Changing roles and responsibilities

C. Learning and adopting complex protocols to manage MS

D. Adjusting to the dynamic nature of the disease

E. Considering the ethnocultural background of each person in the system

F. Realizing that change and complexity are inherent in MS, as in any chronic illness

G. Determining the strategies for change

  1. Accurately assess the patient's status and functioning

  2. Possess clinically relevant technical skills

  3. Collect, analyze, and synthesize data

  4. Jointly, with the patient, develop specific milestones to track patient progress

5. Continuously monitor the quality of care and make appropriate adjustments to the care plan
6. Monitor the delivery of services to the patient with regular communication
7. Identify patient needs and issues during each interaction
8. Assess clinical, social, or other factors influencing the impact on outcomes
9. Assess caregiver or family needs throughout the spectrum of disease
10. Determine the type and level of cultural influences on the patient and family
11. Identify and acknowledge the client's belief or value system
12. Identify potential barriers to client goals or treatment plan
13. Continually reassess plan of care
14. Maintain accurate and detailed records
15. Utilize these concepts to promote sustained adherence to complex protocols

RESOURCES

Curtis, B. T. (2015, September–October). The quintessential nurse activist and change agent. *American Nurse, 47*(5), 13.

Halper, J. (2011). Disease modifying agents and nursing implications. In J. Halper & N. J. Holland (Eds.). *Comprehensive nursing care in multiple sclerosis* (3rd ed.). New York, NY: Springer Publishing Company.

Kline, R. (2013, February 13–19). Stand up and be an agent for change. *Nursing Standard, 27*(24), 16–17.

Lehman, K. L. (2008, July/August). Change management: Magic or mayhem? *Journal for Nurses in Staff Development, 24*(4), 176–184.

Martin, L. R., Haskard-Zolnierek, K. B., & DiMatteo, M. R. (2010). *Health behavior change and treatment adherence.* New York, NY: Oxford University Press.

Ozer, M. O. (2000). *Management of persons with chronic neurologic illness.* Boston, MA: Butterworth Heinemann.

Shapiro, S. E., & Donaldson, N. A. (2008, July/September). Evidence-based practice for advanced practice emergency nurses, part III: Planning, implementing, and evaluating an evidence-based small test of change. *Advanced Emergency Nursing Journal, 30*(3), 222–223.

Wallace, K. A., & Lahti, E. (2005, April/June). Motivation in later life: A psychosocial perspective. *Topics in Geriatric Rehabilitation, 21*(2), 95–106.

4

Multiple Sclerosis Nurses' Code of Professional Conduct

OBJECTIVES

Upon completion of this chapter, the learner will be able to:

- *Define important terms that are essential in the professional practice of health care*
- *Cite principles of professional conduct that guide health care*

A multiple sclerosis (MS) nurse has a moral obligation to sustain high standards of professionalism. The purpose of this obligation is to guide the MS nurse in the practice of MS nursing. This moral obligation is defined as performance of a morally good act or, rather, what ought to be done or should be done. The MS nurse provides care to promote the health and well-being of patients with MS and their families.

Ethical principles that guide the MS nurse are beneficence, nonmaleficence, autonomy, stewardship, and justice.

- **Beneficence:** Moral requirement to promote good
- **Nonmaleficence:** Do no harm
- **Autonomy:** Respect for self-determination

- **Stewardship:** Preserve your own being
- **Justice:** Fair and equitable determination of distribution of resources and fair treatment for individuals and society

GUIDING PRINCIPLES FOR THE MS NURSING PROFESSIONAL

As an MS nursing professional, the nurse:
- Seeks what is good for patients and families
- Recognizes that quality of life is defined by the person with MS
- Recognizes and respects the patient's right to care regardless of age, race, gender, ethnicity, religion, lifestyle, sexual orientation, economic status, or level of disability
- Recognizes the patient's right to MS specialist care
- Promotes impartial treatment
- Recognizes the patient's right to treatment and therapies, including experimental treatments
- Recognizes the patient's right to have access to MS medications
- Knows that patients have the right to be informed and to understand advanced health care directives (living wills and durable powers of attorney) concerning the right to receive resuscitation, refuse appropriate treatment, request do-not-resuscitate orders, or request the discontinuation of life support measures
- Is responsible for providing information to the patient with MS and family to facilitate informed consent for all treatments and procedures
- Participates in research and is aware of the principles of informed consent, the criteria for inclusion and exclusion in research protocols, and the right of the individual to withdraw from a protocol at any time
- Recognizes and maintains the patient's privacy, assuring confidentiality, except when there is a clear, serious, and immediate danger to the patient or others
- Has a moral obligation to offer access to care, cost containment, and quality care
- Affirms that patients with MS have a right to be informed, without bias, coercion, or deception, about treatment options, potential effect, and adverse effects of treatments
- Supports the fact that patients with MS have a right to refuse treatment and continue to receive alternative care
- Recognizes that the patient with MS has a right to review his or her medical record and the right to have information explained
- Requires participation of the patient with MS in an ongoing partnership to develop an effective plan of care, using a process considering diversity, individual autonomy, and responsibility

- Practices competently, consulting and referring when indicated by professional judgment
- Takes appropriate action to protect patients from harm when endangered by incompetent or unethical clinical practice
- Promotes and supports improved practice through professionalism, education, certification, and nursing research
- Promotes local and national efforts to improve public education, legislation to ensure access to quality care, and long-term care initiatives that meet the health needs of patients with MS and their families

RESOURCES

Bandman, E. L., & Bandman, B. (1995). *Nursing ethics through the life span.* Norwalk, CT: Appleton and Lange.

Butts, J. B., & Rich, K. (2005). *Nursing ethics: Across the curriculum and into practice.* Sudbury, MA: Jones & Bartlett Learning.

Byrd, G. D., & Winkelstein, P. (2013, October). A comparative analysis of moral principles and behavioral norms in eight ethical codes relevant to health sciences librarianship, medical informatics, and the health professions. *Journal of the Medical Library Association, 102*(4), 247–256.

Gray, B. (2014, July 4). Bioethics for New Zealand/Aotearoa. *New Zealand Medical Journal, 127*(1397), 67–76.

Griffith, R. (2015, April). Understanding the code: Upholding dignity. *British Journal of Community Nursing, 20*(4), 196–198.

International Organization of Multiple Sclerosis Nurses. (n.d.). Retrieved from www.iomsn.org

Klein, T. (2014, October–December). Philanthropic dilemmas and the nurse administrator role. *Nursing Administration Quarterly, 38*(4), 319–326.

Multiple Sclerosis Trust. (n.d.). Retrieved from www.mstrust.org.uk

Saini, R., Saini, P., & Alagh, P. (2014, May–June). Assessment of knowledge of nurses regarding bioethics. *Nursing Journal of India, 105*(3), 101–104.

Salminen, L., Stolt, M., Metsamaki, R., Rinne, J., Kasen, A., & Leino-Kilpi, H. (2015, July). Ethical principles in the work of nurse educator: A cross sectional study. *Nurse Education Today, 36*, 18–22.

Thompson, I. E., Melia, K. M., & Boyd, K. M. (2006). *Nursing ethics.* Philadelphia, PA: Elsevier Health Sciences.

Tschudin, V. (2003). *Ethics in nursing: The caring relationship.* Philadelphia, PA: Elsevier Health Sciences.

II

The Diagnosis of Multiple Sclerosis

5

Epidemiology of Multiple Sclerosis

OBJECTIVES

Upon completion of this chapter, the learner will be able to:

- Describe the difference between disease incidence and prevalence
- Provide an overview of the epidemiology of multiple sclerosis (MS)
- Discuss the implications of MS epidemiology in patient and family education

- Research into multiple sclerosis (MS) includes epidemiologic inquiries.
- Epidemiology is the study of the natural history of the disease.
- The *incidence* is defined as the number of new cases of the disease beginning in a unit of time within a specified population. This is usually given as an annual incidence rate in cases per 100,000 per year. The date of onset of clinical symptoms decides the time of accession, although, occasionally, the date of first diagnosis is used.
- Prevalence is easier to calculate than incidence because all cases are included regardless of disease duration. Nevertheless, accurate assessment of prevalence is still difficult because of the difficulty of ascertaining when a case is one of full disease.
- The point prevalence rate is more properly called a *ratio* and refers to the number of diagnoses within the community.

- The major clinical criteria in current use for MS are those by the Poser committee and a recent set of criteria that includes cases with monosymptomatic onset proposed by McDonald, which strongly emphasizes MRI findings.

- Kurtzke classified MS prevalence rates into high-, medium-, and low-risk groups. High-risk areas include northern and central Europe, Italy, the northern United States, Canada, southeastern Australia, New Zealand, and parts of the former Soviet Union, with rates greater than 30 per 100,000 population.

- Medium-risk areas (prevalence between 5 and 29 per 100,000) include southern Europe, southern United States, northern Australia, northernmost Scandinavia, much of the north Mediterranean basin, parts of the former Soviet Union, white South Africa, and possibly central South America. Low-risk areas (less than 5 per 100,000) include other areas of Africa and Asia, the Caribbean, Mexico, and possibly northern South America.

- In the United States, states south of the 37th parallel have a lower risk than those north of the parallel.

- As early as the 1920s, it was recognized that the distribution of MS was not uniform. In general, people who reside in temperate climates in economically developed occidental countries tend to have a higher rate of MS.

- In the Northern Hemisphere, a diminishing north–south gradient has been well described.

- In the Southern Hemisphere, the reverse has been reported.

- Numerous reports have been made of "clusters," in which several cases of MS have occurred at a similar point.

FAMILIAL RISKS FOR MS

Up to 2% of people with MS have at least one relative with MS.

Empiric recurrence risks (age adjusted):

MS parent-risk for child 4%

MS person-risk for sibling 4%–5%

MS twin with MS risk for co-twin (fraternal) 3%–5%

MS twin with MS risk for co-twin (identical) 20%–26%

Adapted from Schwartz, Vollmer, and Lee (1999) and Sadovnick et al. 2009.

- MS susceptibility has long been known to vary according to gender. Females are more susceptible than males in a ratio greater than 3:1.

- A review of the literature found that relatives (siblings, first-degree cousins, second-degree cousins) have an increased risk of MS susceptibility.

- Recent studies found a strong correlation for MS susceptibility in monozygotic twin pairs when compared with nontwin MS sibling pairs.

- The average age of onset is 10 to 59 years, with the highest incidence between 20 and 40 years.

- Pregnant women have been followed through their pregnancies and up to 6 months after delivery. A sevenfold decrease in exacerbations is observed during pregnancy, and a sevenfold increased risk occurs during the 6 months after delivery.

- Several autoimmune diseases have been associated with MS. No data strongly link associations, but anecdotal reports exist of relationships to diabetes mellitus, rheumatoid arthritis, myasthenia gravis, and bipolar illness.

- Data are influenced by temporal differences and by differences in health care systems, by neurologic expertise, and even by cultural practices.

- Measures of disease frequency involve a numerator (cases) and a denominator (population at risk). Incidence and death rates refer to new cases and to deaths per unit time and population.

- Prevalence rates refer to cases present at one time per unit population.

- Incidence and prevalence rates are derived from surveys of the disease within certain populations; death rates come from published governmental sources.

- MS has a clear predilection for Whites and Caucasians, but other racial groups share the geographic distributions of the Caucasians, although at lower levels.

- Studies have shown a prevalence in Caucasians rather than in Asians, native Hawaiians, or Blacks living in the same geographic area. Japanese prevalence rates are lowest among those of all industrialized countries.

- The disease is rare in African Blacks but high in Scandinavia and in people of Scandinavian descent.

- Prevalence studies for migrants from high-risk to low-risk areas indicate the age of adolescence to be critical for risk retention, because those older than 15 years who migrate retain the MS risk of their birthplace. Those migrating before the age of 15 years acquire the lower risk of their new residence.

■ Migration data support the idea that MS is ordinarily acquired in early adolescence with a lengthy "incubation" or latent period between disease onset and symptom onset. Susceptibility appears to extend to approximately age 45 years.

■ MS is thought to be the result of an interaction of both genetic and environmental factors, with a theory that susceptibility is under the control of several genes that have yet to be identified.

■ No evidence suggests that MS is transmissible.

■ Genetic factors may be a key to the etiology of MS, but increasing evidence suggests that environmental factors play a significant role.

■ The role of infectious agents as triggering factors has been proposed, but no evidence supports this.

■ Epidemiologic data have resulted in a search for infectious agents that may trigger the disease. These have included the following:

A. Retroviruses

B. Bacteria

■ One theory hypothesizes that an autoimmune process might be triggered by an infectious agent involving *molecular mimicry*, in which the immune system normally reacts to a foreign antigen but also reacts against a component of *self*, namely, myelin.

■ Environmental factors such as smoking and vitamin D are currently under investigation.

RESOURCES

Alonso, A., & Herman, M. A. (2008). Temporal trends in the incidence of multiple sclerosis: A systematic review. *Neurology, 71*, 129–135.

Buckle, G. J., Halper, J., & Rintell, D. J. (2013, December). *Advances in multiple sclerosis primer* [AIMS Monograph]. CMSC (Hackensack, NJ) and the France Foundation (Old Lyme, CT).

Compston, A., Ebers, G., Lassmann, H., McDonald, I., & Wekerle, H. (1998). *McAlpine's multiple sclerosis.* London, UK: Churchill Livingstone.

Dunn, S., & Steinman, L. (2013). The gender gap in multiple sclerosis. *JAMA Neurology, 70*, 634–635.

Ebers, G. C., Arnason, B., Bates, D., & MS Forum Workshop Participants. (1998/1999). *Environmental factors in multiple sclerosis.* Proceedings of the MS Forum Modern Management Workshop, Montreal, Quebec, Canada.

Goris, A., Pauwéls, I., & Dubois, B. (2012). Progress in multiple sclerosis genetics. *Current Genomics, 13*, 646–663.

Gourraud, P. A., McElroy, J. P., Caillier, S. J., Johnson, B. A., Santaniello, A., Hauser, S. L., & Oksenberg, J. R. (2011). Aggregation of multiple sclerosis genetic risk variants in multiple and single case families. *Annals of Neurology*, 69(1), 65–74.

Halper, J., & Holland, N. J. (2011). An overview of multiple sclerosis. In J. Halper & N. J. Holland (Eds.), *Comprehensive nursing care in multiple sclerosis* (pp. 1–16). New York, NY: Springer Publishing Company.

Hansen, T., Skytthe, A., Stenager, F., Petersen, H. C., Brønnum-Hansen, H., & Kyvik, K. O. (2005). Concordance for multiple sclerosis in Danish twins: an update of a nationwide study. *Multiple Sclerosis, 11*, 504–510.

Kesselring. J. (1997). Epidemiology. In J. Kesselring (Ed.), *Multiple sclerosis* (pp. 49–53). Cambridge, UK: Cambridge University Press.

Koch, M., Metz, L., Agrawal, S., & Yong, V. W. (2013). Environmental factors and their regulation of immunity in multiple sclerosis. *Journal of Neurology Science, 324*, 10–16.

Kurtzke, J. F., & Wallin, M. T. (2000). Epidemiology. In J. S. Burks & K. P. Johnson (Eds.), *Multiple sclerosis: Diagnosis, medical management, and rehabilitation* (pp. 49–71). New York, NY: Demos Medical.

Nylander, A., & Hafler, D. (2012). Multiple sclerosis. *Journal of Clinical Investigation, 122*, 1180–1188.

Orton, S. M., Herrera, B. M., Valdar, W., Yee, I. M., Ramagopalan, S. V., Sadovnick, A. D., . . . Canadian Collaborative Study Group. (2006). Sex ratio of multiple sclerosis in Canada: A longitudinal study. *Lancet Neurology, 5*(11), 932–936.

Richards, R. G., Sampson, F. C., Beard, S. M., & Rappenden, P. (2002). A review of the natural history and epidemiology of multiple sclerosis: Implications for resource allocation and health economic models. *Health Technology Assessment, 6*(10), 1–73.

Sadovnick, A.D., Yee, I.M., Guimond, C., Reis, J., Dyment, D. A., & Ebers, G. C. (2009). Age of onset in concordant twins and other relative pairs with multiple sclerosis. *American Journal of Epidemiology*, August 1; 1; 170 (3) 289-296.

Schwartz, C.E., Vollmer, T., & Lee H. (1999). Reliability and validity of two self report measures of impairment and disability for MS. *Neurology*, 52(1) 63-70.

Weinshenker, B. G. (1996). Epidemiology of multiple sclerosis. *Neurology Clinics, 14*(2), 291–308.

Weinshenker, B. G., Bass, B., Rice, G. P., Noseworthy, J., Carriere, W., Baskerville, J., & Ebers, G. C. (1989). The natural history of multiple sclerosis: A geographically based study. I. Clinical course and disability. *Brain, 112*(Pt. I), 133–146.

6

The Complete Neurologic Examination

OBJECTIVES

Upon completion of this chapter, the learner will be able to:

- *Describe key components of a neurologic examination*
- *Discuss specific findings related to multiple sclerosis (MS)*
- *Cite the importance of patient and family education during this process*

■ Patient assessment

   A. In assessment, we seek to answer the question "What does this finding mean to the person?"

   B. We ask the following questions:

     1. Why am I doing this assessment?

     2. What is the aim of this assessment?

     3. When should I assess?

     4. What other information will I need?

     5. How will I judge what this information means?

- Taking the history
  A. The first and most important step in a focused assessment is gathering a detailed and accurate history in chronologic order.
  B. Family members or significant others may help contribute information.
  C. While taking the history, appraise the patient's conversational style. Is it coherent? Is the language fluent? Is the language appropriate for the level of education?
  D. Assess level of consciousness, orientation memory, intellectual status, and speech.

- Mental status
  A. The mental status assesses the following:
    1. Orientation to time: "What is the date today?"
    2. Registration: "Listen carefully. I am going to say three words, and you repeat them to me after I stop."
    3. Naming: "What is this?" (Point to a pencil or pen.)
    4. Reading: "Please read this, and do what it says." (Show the words on the stimulus form "Close your eyes.")
    5. The total score is a sum of all the 11 evaluations. Each evaluation is scored with regard to the number of tasks performed correctly. For example, if a patient is able to correctly recall only two of the three objects, a score of 2 is given. A mental status score of less than 20 points out of a maximum of 30 indicates a cognitive deficit.

(*Comment:* The mental status examination is generally used in neurology. For cognitive changes in multiple sclerosis (MS), there are more specific tests used to determine specific deficits related to MS. Description is beyond the scope of this chapter.)

- Cranial nerves
  A. CNI: Olfactory nerve involves assessment of the sense of smell.
  B. CNII: Optic nerve involves assessment of visual acuity and gross visual fields as well as an ophthalmoscopic examination.
  C. CNIII: Pupillary constriction elicited by shining a light into each eye. Each pupil should constrict directly and consensually (constriction of the opposite pupil). A pupillary difference (anisocoria) up to 20% may be preexisting and normal. This nerve also innervates the extraocular muscles that affect lateral and vertical gaze and is tested with CNIV and CNVI. CNIV innervates the superior oblique muscle and aids in the movement of the eye and looking downward and inward. CNVI innervates the lateral rectus muscle of the eye (abduction) in horizontal movement. Testing these three nerves involves testing the extraocular eye movements (nystagmus and isolated paralysis).

D. CNV: Trigeminal nerve has both sensory and motor functions. Sensation of the face and the muscles of mastication are controlled by CNV. Trigeminal neuralgia is a common problem in MS and occurs when this nerve is affected.

E. CNVII: Both motor and sensory components. The motor portion innervates the muscles of the face and scalp; the sensory portion supplies the sense of taste on the anterior two-thirds of the tongue and sensation to the ear canal and behind the ear.

F. CNVIII: Acoustic nerve, which involves hearing and influences equilibrium.

G. CNIX: Supplies sensory sensation to the pharynx, tonsils, and posterior two-thirds of the tongue.

H. CNX: Vagus nerve; it is involved in the gag reflex and is tested with CNIX. It provides motor control to palate, larynx, and pharynx.

I. CNXI: Controls the movement of the sternocleidomastoid and trapezius muscles of the neck and shoulders.

J. CNXII: Motor nerve of the tongue.

- Motor assessment
  A. Motor assessment techniques test muscle innervation by spinal nerves.
  B. Biceps involve elbow flexion and originate at C5 and C6.
  C. Triceps involve elbow extension and originate at C7 to T1.
  D. Rectus abdominis involves trunk flexion and originates at T6 to L1.
  E. Iliopsoas involves hip flexion and originates at L1 to L3.
  F. Quadriceps involves knee extension and originates at L2 to L4.
  G. Biceps femoris involve knee flexion and originate at L5 to S2.
  H. Evaluation of arm drift is a sensitive test for weakness in the upper extremities.
  I. Other sensitive tests for extremity weakness include hand grasp, plantar flexion of the foot, and dorsiflexion of the foot.
  J. Atrophy: Observe large muscle groups for symmetry and determine whether their size is appropriate for the person's age.
  K. Tone: Observe and test muscles for flaccidity, spasticity, or rigidity. Rigidity presents as stiffness regardless of the rate of passive movement. When an extremity is rigid, it "catches" during passive movement.
  L. Spasticity depends on the rate of movement. When the spastic extremity is moved slowly, the tone appears normal. If the extremity is moved quickly, it "catches" and loses all resistance. Does it lose resistance or become resistant?

SUMMARY OF CRANIAL NERVE FUNCTION

Nerve	Function
I—Olfactory	Smell
II—Optic	Vision
III—Oculomotor	Eye movement, pupil contraction, accommodation, and eyelid movement
IV—Trochlear	Down and in movement of eye
V—Trigeminal	Facial sensation, chewing
VI—Abducens	Lateral gaze
VII—Facial	Facial muscles, taste on anterior two-thirds of tongue, and corneal reflex
VIII—Acoustic	Hearing and balance
IX—Glosso-medulla	Taste, swallowing, gag reflex, and cough
X—Vagus	Parasympathetic to organs, laryngeal muscles, speech, and swallowing
XI—Accessory	Movement of head and shoulders
XII—Hypoglossal	Tongue muscles

- Sensory examination
  A. Basic sensory examination consists of pain, light touch, proprioception, stereognosis, and vibration.
    1. Proprioception measures posterior column defects (position of toe—up or down, etc.).
    2. Stereognosis depends on touch and position sense (identification of a familiar object in one's hand).
    3. Vibration sense is tested by placing a vibrating tuning fork over the distal interphalangeal joint of a finger and the great toe.

- Cerebellum and gait
  A. The cerebellum organizes and coordinates movements, but does not control individual muscles. Smooth, coordinated movements depend on the normal functioning of the cerebellum. *Ataxia* describes disorganized, unsteady, or inaccurate movements.
  B. Tests include finger to nose, heel–knee–shin, the Romberg test, and gait assessment.

■ Reflexes

A. The major deep tendon reflexes are as follows:

1. Achilles (S1, S2)

2. Patellar (L3, L4)

3. Biceps (C5, C6)

4. Triceps reflexes (C7, C8)

5. Grading is on a scale from 0 to 5+. Zero reflects no contraction (absent reflex), 1+ is diminished but present, 2+ is normal, 3+ is increased, 4+ is hyperactive with clonus, and 5+ is sustained clonus

6. Asymmetric reflexes indicate neurologic (or muscular) dysfunction

■ Cerebellar disorders

A. Ataxia: Awkwardness of posture and gait; tendency to fall to the same side as the cerebella lesion; poor coordination of movement; overshooting the goal in reaching for an object (dysmetria); inability to perform rapid alternating movements (dysdiadochokinesia), such as finger tapping; scanning speech due to awkward use of speech muscles, resulting in irregularly spaced sounds.

B. Decreased tendon reflexes on the affected side.

C. Asthenia: Muscles tire more easily than normal.

D. Tremor: Usually an intention tremor (evident during purposeful movements).

E. Nystagmus.

■ Miscellaneous notes

A. The left visual field falls on the right half of each retina; the superior visual field falls on the inferior retina. The left visual field projects to the right side of the brain and vice versa.

B. The superior visual field projects below the calcarine fissure in the occipital lobe.

C. A lesion of the medial longitudinal fasciculus, which connects CNIII and CNVI, results in impaired adduction of the ipsilateral eye and nystagmus in abduction of the contralateral eye.

D. *Nystagmus* is a repetitive, tremor-like oscillating movement of the eyes. The most common form is horizontal jerk nystagmus, in which the eyes repetitively move slowly toward one side and then quickly back. Vertical nystagmus is always abnormal, signifying a disorder in brain stem function.

SIGNIFICANT FINDINGS INDICATIVE OF MULTIPLE SCLEROSIS

Sign	CNS Location
Partial list of ocular motor findings in MS	
Opsoclonus	Cerebellum
Nystagmus	Cerebellum
Saccadic dysmetria	cerebellum, brain stem
INO	MLF
Partial list of cranial nerve dysfunction in MS	
Hemianopsia	CNII
Ptosis	CNIII
Upward–outward gaze deviation	CNIV
Trigeminal neuralgia	CNV
Disruption of abduction of eye	CNVI
Weakness, facial muscles	CNVII
Hearing loss, tinnitus, vertigo	CNVIII
Dysphagia, dysarthria	CNIX
Decreased phonation, diminished gag	CNX
Weakness shoulder shrug	CNXI
Tongue weakness	CNXII

INO, internuclear ophthalmoplegia; MLF, medial longitudinal fasciculus; MS, multiple sclerosis.

E. Pendular nystagmus, in which one eye moves at equal speeds in both directions, commonly is congenital.

F. Intranuclear ophthalmoplegia—The affected eye, which should turn inward, cannot move past the midline; that is, the affected eye looks straight ahead. As the other eye turns outward, it often makes involuntary, repetitive fluttering movements called *nystagmus,* that is, the eye rapidly moves in one direction, then slowly drifts in the other direction. In young people, bilateral intranuclear ophthalmoplegia is associated with a diagnosis of MS.

G. Doll's eye phenomenon occurs when the head is turned suddenly to one side. Normally, there is a tendency for the eyes to lag behind. This reflex is believed to be brain stem mediated, and any asymmetry or lack of response is believed to reflect significant brain stem dysfunction.

■ Implications for patient and family education

A. It is important to explain significant findings to the patient and/ or family. Keep explanations simple, and use graphics and written explanations when appropriate. Linking clinical care to neurologic findings and associated symptoms is an important educational function for the MS nursing professional and helps to restore a sense of control to the patient.

RESOURCES

Bhidayashiri, R., Waters, M. F., & Giza, C. C. (2005). *Neurological differential diagnosis*. Malden, MA: Blackwell.

Costello, K., & Harris, C. (2009). *Diagnosing multiple sclerosis* [CD ROM]. IOMSN.

Costello, K., & Morgante, L. (2004). *Neurologic examination for the MS nurse* [CD ROM]. IOMSN.

Giesser, B. G. (2011). *Primer on multiple sclerosis*. New York, NY: Oxford University Press.

Murray, T. A., Kelly, N. R., & Jenkins, S. (2002). The complete neurological examination: What every nurse practitioner should know. *Advance Nurse Practitioners, 10*(7), 24–30.

Pittock, S. J. (2010). Clinical features and natural history of multiple sclerosis: The nature of the beast. In C. F. Lucchinetti & R. Hohlfeld (Eds.), *Multiple sclerosis 3* (1st ed., pp. 1–18). Philadelphia, PA: Saunders Elsevier.

7

Magnetic Resonance Imaging

OBJECTIVES

Upon completion of this chapter, the learner will be able to:

- Describe the role of MRI in the diagnosis, treatment, and monitoring of multiple sclerosis (MS)
- Discuss MRI in relation to disease-modifying therapies
- Cite the use of MRI in MS research
- Differentiate current and emerging neuroimaging techniques

- Basic overview of MRI
  - A. Magnetic resonance imaging is commonly referred to as MRI.
  - B. Unlike computed axial tomography scans, MRI does not use x-rays to create pictures of the body.
  - C. The technology uses a complicated array of physics, mathematics, and high-performance computing techniques.
  - D. An MRI scanner consists of a very large and very strong, but harmless, magnet; the patient lies within the magnet's field.
  - E. The scanner generates pictures by analyzing how water molecules react to electrical impulses in this strong magnetic environment.

    F. This involves radio frequency waves.

    G. Newer and more advanced techniques are available or under development.

      1. MTI or magnetization transfer imaging

      2. MRS or magnetic resonance spectroscopy

■ MRI principles

    A. MRI images are based upon the water content in normal and abnormal tissues.

    B. When a person lies in the magnetic field on an MR unit, hydrogen (water) protons align with the axis of the magnet.

    C. A radio frequency pulse is transmitted, rotating the protons.

    D. When the pulse is turned off, the protons return to their previous states.

    E. The return to alignment is known as *relaxation.*

    F. Measurement of the energy released with the movement of protons provides the MRI images. When and how the signal is captured provide different images known as T1, T2, proton density, or fluid attenuated inversion recovery (FLAIR).

      1. FLAIR imaging generates images where water appears dark rather than bright on T2-weighted scans.

    G. Multiple sclerosis (MS) lesions are evident on MRI images because of free water associated with edema and inflammation and because of tissue destruction.

      1. On T1 images, MS lesions may appear dark, an appearance felt to be associated with axonal disruption and destruction.

        a. Acute lesions may appear dark on T1 for a short period.

        b. Lesions that continue to appear dark are thought to be associated with permanent damage.

      2. On T2 images, MS lesions appear white, similar to the appearance of spinal fluid. T2 images show both new and chronic lesions, and measurement of the number of T2 lesions is considered "disease burden."

      3. Gadolinium (Gd) contrast is used to demonstrate areas of acute inflammation.

        a. Gd is not able to cross an intact blood–brain barrier (BBB).

        b. Areas of acute inflammation in MS occur because of breakdown of the BBB and migration of inflammatory immune system cells into the brain parenchyma.

        c. When breakdown of the BBB occurs, GD delivered intravenously during an MRI is able to cross the BBB and create enhancement on T1 scans, causing acute lesions to appear bright white.

H. Pulse sequences used for MRI are known as *spin echo*.

I. MS scans include the entire brain and at times the spinal cord, although MS lesions are most frequent in the periventricular region.

■ Uses of MRI in MS

A. The primary use of MRI in MS is to confirm the diagnosis and rule out other possible conditions.

B. Early in the disease process, MRI seems to be moderately correlated with later disability. The earlier lesions are seen on MRI, the earlier disability progression appears.

C. MRI may also be used to monitor the effectiveness of drugs in clinical trials.

D. MRI lesions may precede overt symptoms, as seen in studies of the natural history of MS.

E. MRI has provided valuable insights into the course of the illness and has helped to identify new therapies that have at least a partial effect on disease activity.

F. Under the new diagnostic criteria proposed by McDonald et al., T2-weighted lesions in the periventricular white matter, brain stem, and spinal cord, and Gd enhancement on T1 imaging, along with hypointensities (black holes) on T1 images, support the diagnosis of MS.

■ Diagnosis of MS is based on two episodes of neurologic symptoms referable to the central nervous system separated in space (different locations in the central nervous system) or dissemination in space (DIS) and time (different point in time for each event) or dissemination in time (DIT). In the revised 2010 McDonald criteria, DIT can be shown by a new T2 and/or gadolinium-enhancing lesion(s) on follow-up MRI, with reference to a baseline scan, irrespective of the timing of the baseline MR or simultaneous presence of asymptomatic gadolinium-enhancing and nonenhancing lesions at any time.

■ The evolution of the MS lesion

A. Disruption of the BBB occurs, with inflammation.

B. Gd enhancement occurs at active sites.

C. This enhancement usually subsides in 3 to 6 weeks, leaving a "white spot" on the MRI image.

D. Sometimes, these areas become larger and reinflamed with new disease activity, and then once again subside.

E. Over time, repeated inflammation may cause extensive damage within the lesion.

1. These may appear as hypointense lesions on T1 images, also known as *black holes*.

F. New MRI lesions can be "clinically silent." Several factors influence whether a lesion visible on MRI correlates with an overt clinical sign or symptom. These are as follows:

1. Location of the lesion

2. Number of lesions

3. Severity of the damage

G. In the relapsing–remitting phase, a great deal of MRI activity occurs.

H. In the secondary progressive phase, more symptoms are present, and less new MRI activity occurs; fewer acute inflamed lesions are present and more chronic, older lesions that reflect irreversible axonal damage and atrophy. MRI activity may fall off because less inflammatory activity is occurring.

I. MRI guidelines developed through an expert consensus committee of the Consortium of Multiple Sclerosis Centers recommend that MRI be used as part of the diagnosis of MS (www.mscare.org).

1. There is no current recommendation for MRIs to be done at preset intervals throughout the lifetime of the disease

2. Repeat MRI is appropriate if there is a change in condition of the patient or a change in treatment is considered

- Various MRI techniques currently in the research arena may provide more information about MS, including effects on the normal-appearing white matter.

A. MR spectroscopy

B. Diffusion tensor imaging

C. Magnetization transfer

- Other imaging techniques illustrate the plasticity of the brain after injury

A. Functional MRI or fMRI

1. Demonstrates functional reorganization

- It is likely that this technology will play a larger role in the long-term management of MS. An international panel recently updated the diagnostic criteria for MS (Polman et al., 2010), simplifying MRI evidence for DIS and DIT. Other technologies, such as magnetization transfer MRI and MRS, have been applied to the evaluation of patients with MS. Magnetization transfer changes may reflect changes in myelin, although edema may also contribute to changes. MRS can detect changes in metabolites.

GLOSSARY

- *Black hole—Chronic T1-hypointense lesions that reflect severe demyelination, axonal loss, and matrix destruction.*

- *Clinical MRI paradox—the presence of new lesions on MRI in the absence of clinical symptoms and clinical progression in the absence of new MRI lesions.*

- *Gd—a chemical compound that can be administered to a person during MRI to help distinguish between new and old lesions.*

- *Juxtacortical—adjacent to white matter.*

- *T1 relaxation time—time required for protons to realign within the magnetic field.*

- *T1-weighted images—show acute MS lesions as hypointense because of edema of the damaged brain tissue.*

- *T2 lesion load—total lesion number and/or volume.*

- *T2-weighted images—show hyperintense bright lesions representing demyelination, edema, gliosis, or matrix destruction.*

RESOURCES

Bakshi, R., Thompson, A. J., Rocca, M. A., Pelletier, D., Dousset, V., Barkhof, F., . . . Filippi, M. (2008). MRI in multiple sclerosis: Current status and future prospects. *Lancet Neurology, 7*, 615–625.

Clanet, M., & Bates, D. (Eds.). (1997). *Imaging in multiple sclerosis* [MS Forum]. Berlin, Germany: Schering.

CMSC 2008 Guidelines for use of MRI in MS. (2009). Retrieved from www.mscare.org

Confavreaux, C. V., Vukusic, S., & Adeleine, P. (2003). Early predictors and progression of irreversible disability in multiple sclerosis. *Brain, 126,* 770–782.

Consortium of MS Centers. (2015). *Revised recommendations for a standard MRI protocol and clinical guidelines for the diagnosis and follow-up of multiple sclerosis* Hackensack, NJ: Author.

Cook, S. D. (Ed.). (2001). *The multiple sclerosis handbook.* New York, NY: Marcel Dekker.

Fazekas, F., Soelberg-Sorensen, P., Comi, G., & Filippi, M. (2007). MRI to monitor treatment efficacy in multiple sclerosis. *Journal of Neuroimaging, 17*(Suppl. 1), 505–555.

Filippi, M., Rocca, M. A., Arnold, D. L., Bakshi, R., Barkhof, F., De Stefano, N., . . . Wolinsky, J. S. (2006). EFNS guidelines on the use of neuroimaging in the management of multiple sclerosis. *European Journal of Neurology, 13*(4), 313–325.

Hawkins, C., & Wolinsky, J. S. (2000). *Principles of treatments in multiple sclerosis.* Oxford, UK: Butterworth-Heinemann.

Li, D. K., Li, M. J., Traboulsee, A., Zhao, G., Riddehough, A., & Paty, D. (2006). The use of MRI as an outcome measure in clinical trials. *Advances in Neurology, 98,* 203–226.

McDonald, W. I., Compston, A., Edan, G., Goodkin, D., Hartung, H. P., Lublin, F. D., . . . Wolinsky, J. S. (2001). Recommended diagnostic criteria for multiple sclerosis. *Annals of Neurology, 50,* 121–127.

Miller, A., Johnson, K. P., Lublin, F., Murray, T. J., Whitaker, J. N., & Wolinsky, J. S. (Eds.). (2002). *MRI in the management of MS*. Beechwood, OH: Current Therapeutics.

Neuroimaging in multiple sclerosis (a DVD for MS nurses). (2011). Retrieved from www.iomsn.org

Palace, J. (2001). Making the diagnosis of multiple sclerosis. *Journal of Neurology, Neurosurgery and Psychiatry, 71*(Suppl.), ii3–ii8.

Polman, C. H., Reingold, S. C., Banwell, B., Clanet, M., Cohen, J. A., Filippi, M., . . . Wolinsky, J. S. (2011). Diagnostic criteria for multiple sclerosis: 2010 revisions to the "McDonald criteria." *Annals of Neurology, 69,* 292–302.

Polman, C. H., Reingold, S. C., Edan, G., Filippi, M., Hartung, H. P., Kappos, L., . . . Wolinsky, J. S. (2005). Diagnostic criteria for multiple sclerosis: 2005 revisions to the "McDonald criteria." *Annals of Neurology, 58,* 840–846.

Rovira, A., & Leon, A. (2008). MR in the diagnosis and monitoring of multiple sclerosis: An overview. *European Journal of Radiology, 67,* 409–414.

Simon, J. H. (2000). Magnetic resonance imaging in the diagnosis of multiple sclerosis, elucidation of disease course, and determining prognosis. In J. Burks & K. Johnson (Eds.), *Multiple sclerosis diagnosis, medical management, and rehabilitation* (pp. 100–101). New York, NY: Demos Medical.

Simon, J. H., Li, D., Traboulsee, A., Coyle, P. K., Arnold, D. L., Barkhof, F., . . . Wolinsky, J. S. (2006). Standardized MR imaging protocol for multiple sclerosis: Consortium of MS Centers consensus guidelines. *American Journal of Neuroradiology, 27*(2), 455–461.

Thompson, A. J., Polman, C. H., Miller, D. H., McDonald, W. I., Brochet, B., Filippi, M., & De Sá, J. (1997). Primary progressive multiple sclerosis. *Brain, 120*(6), 1085–1096.

Wolinsky, J. S. (2007). The multiple sclerosis disease process as characterized by magnetic resonance imaging. In J. A. Cohen & R. A. Rudick (Eds.), *Multiple sclerosis therapeutics* (3rd ed., pp. 45–63). London: UK: Informa Healthcare.

Zivadinov, R., Stosic, M., Cox, J. L., Ramasamy, D. P., & Dwyer, M. G. (2008). The place of conventional MRI and newly emerging MRI techniques in monitoring different aspects of treatment outcome. *Journal of Neurology, 255*(Suppl. 1), 61–74.

8

The Diagnosis and Prognosis of Multiple Sclerosis

OBJECTIVES

Upon completion of this chapter, the learner will be able to:

- Describe the pathophysiology of multiple sclerosis (MS)
- Describe common symptoms of MS
- Discuss the diagnostic process in MS
- Cite the common disease courses seen in MS, including clinically isolated syndrome (CIS)
- Identify common laboratory tests used in the diagnostic process

Multiple sclerosis (MS) is a clinical diagnosis because no definitive laboratory test exists. It is common practice to perform a battery of pertinent investigations to exclude other conditions and to provide objective evidence that MS is the correct diagnosis. This also enables the neurologist to create a prognostic profile to guide therapeutic choices.

- Pathophysiology of MS
    - A. The etiology of MS is not known.
    - B. The most widely believed hypothesis is that it is a virus-induced immune-mediated disease.

C. A great deal of effort has gone into attempts to understand the immunology of MS using the animal model, experimental autoimmune encephalomyelitis.

D. For normal nerve fibers, the myelin sheath has a uniform thickness, and myelin segments between nodes of Ranvier (internodal segments) are of uniform length except near the end of each fiber, where internodes become progressively shorter.

E. The pathology of MS consists of lesions disseminated in location and of varying age. Lesions are present in both white and gray matter, but the gray matter lesions are less evident on casual inspection. Oligodendrocytes are damaged in the MS disease process.

F. Lesions range from acute plaques with active inflammatory infiltrates and macrophages loaded with lipid and myelin degeneration products to chronic, inactive, demyelinated scars.

G. Slowed conduction and conduction failure occur in demyelinated fibers. Conduction failure is due to fiber fatigue or to an increase in body temperature or both.

H. Ongoing inflammation, demyelination, and scarring ultimately result in irreversible axonal damage and loss.

I. Acute MS lesions are characterized by T lymphocytes, plasma cells, macrophages, and bare, demyelinated, or transected axons.

J. Brain atrophy in MS is widely recognized and represents a negative pathologic change. It may develop as an early measure of disease progression, and its slowing may be used as a measure of therapy efficacy in long-term management.

■ Demographics of MS

A. Most patients are young women who present with symptoms of episodic neurologic problems that spontaneously improve. Worldwide data suggest that twice as many women get MS as men.

B. The less common presentation is an older man or woman who has gradual development of neurologic deficits. Most often, this takes the form of a progressive myelopathy.

C. Seventy to seventy-five percent of patients with MS are female.

D. The only exception to this is in primary progressive MS, in which an equal gender ratio exists.

E. Most patients with MS are Caucasian.

F. MS is rare among Africans, Asians, and Native Americans.

G. African Americans have levels of MS consistent with the mixing of the gene pool.

H. Asians are more likely to have optic and spinal cord nerve involvement. This type of MS has an older age onset, fewer brain lesions on MRI, and more enhancing lesions in the spinal cord.

I. The average age of onset is 28 to 30 years.

J. Fewer than 1% of patients have an onset before the age of 10 years; before age of 16 years, the onset is 1.2% to 6%.

■ Prognostic factors in MS

A. Positive predictors in MS include the following:

   1. Younger age at onset

   2. Female gender

   3. Normal MRI at presentation

   4. Complete recovery from first relapse

   5. Low relapse rate

   6. Long interval to second relapse

   7. Low disability at 2 and 4 years

B. Unfavorable predictors in MS include the following:

   1. Older age at onset

   2. Male gender

   3. High lesion load on MRI at presentation

   4. Lack of recovery from first relapse

   5. High relapse rate

   6. Early cerebellar involvement

   7. Short interval to second relapse

   8. Early development of mild disability

   9. Insidious motor onset

■ Clinical profile of MS

A. Requires symptomatic disease over time, confirmed by objective evidence on neurologic examination. *Symptomatic disease* means neurologic worsening in the form of episodic attacks or slow progression.

B. The most common presentations are as follows:

   1. Sensory disturbance such as numbness, paresthesias, pain, or Lhermitte's sign (electric shock sensations or paresthesias that extend down the back and into the legs or arms elicited by neck flexion; 21%–55% of patients):

      a. Often begins in the limbs and migrates proximally

      b. Tingling

    c. Lhermitte's sign

    d. Neuritic pain

    e. Diminished vibratory sensation

    f. Impaired position sense

    g. Useless hand syndrome

2. Motor abnormalities:

    a. Corticospinal (32%–41%)

    b. Heaviness, weakness, abnormal deep tendon reflexes (DTRs)

    c. Positive Babinski response

    d. Spastic limb weakness

3. Visual problems:

    a. Brain stem

    b. Eye movement abnormalities (diplopia nystagmus, internuclear ophthalmoplegia)

    c. Optic neuritis (in up to 25% of patients)

4. Cerebellar gait ataxia and limb tremor.

C. Laboratory testing is used to help document that no alternative disorders explain the neurologic picture and that a pattern of central nervous system (CNS) lesion involvement is consistent with MS, with no white matter involvement.

1. Previous diagnostic criteria (Schumacher and Poser) have been supplemented by new criteria for a clinically isolated syndrome (CIS) to allow an MRI-supported diagnosis.

2. The newer McDonald criteria, proposed in 2001 and revised in 2010 (www.nmss.org, 2010 revision to the McDonald criteria):

    a. Developed by a large international committee funded by the National Multiple Sclerosis Society and the Multiple Sclerosis International Federation to revise criteria to include new technology

    b. Preserves traditional diagnostic criteria of two attacks of disease separated in space and time

    c. Must be no better explanation

    d. Adds MRI, cerebrospinal fluid (CSF), and evoked potentials (EP) criteria

    e. Three possible outcomes after workup:

        i. Multiple sclerosis

        ii. Possible MS

        iii. Not MS

    f. Monosymptomatic presentation:

       i. One attack

      ii. One objective clinical lesion

     iii. MRI evidence

    g. Primary progressive MS:

       i. Positive CSF and dissemination in space

      ii. MRI evidence along with EP and CSF

     iii. Continued progression over 1 year

    h. Although MRI is recognized as an invaluable tool, it is not appropriate to use it in isolation; diagnosis should always be made in the clinical context

    i. Paraclinical evidence along with MRI includes cerebrospinal fluid with immunoglobulin G (IgG) oligoclonal bands or intrathecal IgG production

    j. Evoked potential tests are used to document lesions disseminated in space to provide objective evidence to document subjective complaints or to confirm a pattern of CNS involvement consistent with MS. Nerve conduction is studied in the visual tracts, in the brain stem, and through the spinal cord (visual evoked potential, VEP; brain stem auditory evoked potential, BAEP; and sensory evoked potential, SEP).

■ Immunology of MS

  A. The evidence for immune system involvement in MS is fairly clear, whereas evidence that it is an autoimmune disease is more indirect.

  B. People with MS seem to have clear-cut abnormalities in immune function.

    1. Unusually high reactivity of immune system T cells to proteins of myelin in the CNS (termed *antigens,* since they can trigger immune responses)

    2. An overrepresentation of cells that enhance immune responses (pro-inflammatory T helper cells)

    3. A relative underrepresentation of cells that suppress immune responses (suppressor T cells)

    4. The presence of immune system cells in MS lesions in the brain, spinal cord, and optic nerves

    5. Recently, the role of B lymphocytes that are responsible for producing antibodies has been emphasized

Table 8.1 Principal Differential Diagnosis of MS

Type of cause	Disorder or causative agent
Infection	Lyme disease, syphilis, progressive multifocal leukoencephalopathy, HIV, HTLV-1
Inflammatory	Systemic lupus erythematosus, Sjögren's syndrome, vasculitis, sarcoidosis, Behcet's disease
Metabolic	Vitamin B_{12} deficiency, lysosomal disorders, adrenoleukodystrophy, mitochondrial disorders, other genetic disorders
Neoplasm	CNS lymphoma
Spine disease	Degenerative spinal disease, vascular malformation

CNS, central nervous system; HIV, human immunodeficiency virus; HTLV-1, human T-cell leucopenia virus; MS, multiple sclerosis.

Reprinted with permission from Burks & Johnson (2000).

DIFFERENTIAL DIAGNOSIS OF MS

- *HIV, human immunodeficiency virus; PML, progressive multifocal leukoencephalopathy; HTLV, human T-cell leucopenia virus; SLE, systemic lupus erythematosus.*

Source: Cohen & Rensel (2000).

---

6. "Direct" evidence that MS is an autoimmune disease is difficult to obtain in humans, but in the animal model (experimental autoimmune encephalomyelitis) it is clear

- Many studies during the latter part of the 20th century increased our understanding of the immune system's reactivity to myelin in MS, including specificity immune responses to myelin antigens.

- Etiology of MS

   A. The genetic link in MS is borne out by the facts that:

   1. An increased susceptibility is present in certain families in which MS already occurs

   2. A high genetic susceptibility is observed in monozygotic twins (20%–40%)

   3. Some genetically isolated ethnic groups never develop MS (Hutterites in Canada; East-European gypsies)

4. The racial differences in MS prevalence are likely to be genetically based

5. Although genetics plays a role in MS susceptibility, the nature of the link is both complex and largely unknown

6. Great interest exists in environmental triggering factors. Over the decades, studies have been made of retroviral (HTLV-1, HHV6, and canine distemper) and bacterial (e.g., *Chlamydia pneumoniae*) triggers

7. Evidence is anecdotal at this point, with no substantiation in research

■ Clinical subtypes of MS (disease courses)

A. Primary progressive MS involves slow worsening from onset and is considered to be a single attack. Patients with primary progressive MS may have to be observed over time; 15% of people with MS show this pattern.

B. Patients with relapsing–remitting MS experience neurologic attacks with variable recovery, but are clinically stable between attacks. Among this group are a minority of patients who will have minimal disease activity and little or no disability 25 years into their disease. These patients have benign or mild MS and may comprise 10% to 20% of those with MS.

C. Secondary progressive MS is the major progressive form of the disease and accounts for approximately 30% of all patients with MS. These patients start with relapsing–remitting disease, then slowly begin to worsen.

D. By 10 years, 50%, and by 20 to 15 years, at least 80% of untreated relapsing patients will become secondary progressive.

E. An additional term in the literature, *transitional MS*, refers to those patients who are evolving into the secondary progressive stage.

F. Some patients begin with no attacks and a progressive course and, later in their disease, begin having exacerbations (progressive-relapsing).

G. CISs are monoregional acute monophasic syndromes that encompass optic neuritis, transverse myelitis, isolated brain stem, or cerebellar syndromes. These patients have a high risk of MS, as confirmed by recent studies. MRI scans with T2 lesions predict a greater than 80% conversion to MS within 10 years.

H. In 2013, reexamination of MS-disease phenotypes by the International Advisory Committee on Clinical Trials refined descriptors that included consideration of disease activity (based on clinical relapse rate and imaging findings) and disease progression.

I. They categorized CIS and relapsing–remitting MS (R–RMS) as active, and not active; primary progressive MS (PPMS) and secondary progressive MS (SPMS) as active with progression, active without progression, not active with progression, and not active without progression.

■ Red flags in the diagnosis of MS

    A. One should be concerned about patients who:

       1. Have not had any laboratory tests

       2. Have normal neurologic examinations and normal laboratory studies

       3. Have only peripheral nerve involvement

       4. Have disease onset at a very early or very late age

RESOURCES

Burks, J. S., & Johnson, K. P. (2000). *Multiple sclerosis: Diagnosis, medical management, and rehabilitation.* New York, NY: Demos Medical.

Cohen, J., & Rensel, M. (2000). The differential diagnosis and clues to misdiagnosis. In J. Burks & K. Johnson (Eds.), *Multiple sclerosis: Diagnosis, medical management and rehabilitation* (pp. 127–138). New York, NY: Demos Medical.

Confavreaux, C., & Vukusic, S. (2006). Natural history of multiple sclerosis: A unifying concept. *Brain, 129,* 606–616.

Coyle, P. K. (2000). Diagnosis and classification of inflammatory demyelinating disorders. In J. S. Burks & K. P. Johnson (Eds.), *Multiple sclerosis: Diagnosis, medical management, and rehabilitation* (pp. 81–97). New York, NY: Demos Medical.

Halper, J. (2007). The nature of multiple sclerosis. In *Advanced concepts in multiple sclerosis nursing care* (2nd ed.). New York, NY: Demos Medical.

Hawkins, C., & Wolinsky, J. S. (2000). *Principles of treatments in multiple sclerosis.* Oxford, UK: Butterworth-Heinemann.

Lublin, D., Reingold, S. C., Cohen, J. A., Cutter, G. R., Sorenson, P. S., Thompson, A. J., . . . Polman, C. H. (2014). Defining the clinical course of multiple sclerosis. *Neurology, 83*(3), 278–286.

Martin, R., & Dhib-Jalbut, S. (2000). Immunology and etiologic concepts. In J. S. Burks & K. P. Johnson (Eds.), *Multiple sclerosis: Diagnosis, medical management, and rehabilitation* (pp. 141–165). New York, NY: Demos Medical.

McDonald, W. I., Compston, A., Edan, G., Goodkin, D., Hartung, H. P., Lublin, F. D., . . . Wolinsky, J. S. (2001). Recommended diagnostic criteria for multiple sclerosis: Guidelines from the International Panel on the Diagnosis of Multiple Sclerosis. *Annals of Neurology, 50,* 121–127.

Palace, J. (2001). Making the diagnosis of multiple sclerosis. *Journal of Neurology, Neurosurgery and Psychiatry, 71*(Suppl. 2), ii3–ii8.

Polman, C. H., Reingold, S. C., Banwell, B., Clanet, M., Cohen, J. A., Filippi, M., . . . Wolinsky, J. S. (2011). Diagnostic criteria for multiple sclerosis: 2010 revisions to the "McDonald Criteria." *Annals of Neurology, 69*, 292–302.

Polman, C. H., Reingold, S. C., Edan, G., Filippi, M., Hartung, H. P., Kappos, L., . . . Wolinsky, J. S. (2005). Diagnostic criteria for multiple sclerosis: 2005 revisions to the "McDonald Criteria." *Annals of Neurology, 58*(6), 840–846.

Thompson, A. J., Polman, C. H., Miller, D. H., McDonald, W. I., Brochet, B., Filippi, M., & De Sá, J. (1997). Primary progressive multiple sclerosis. *Brain, 120*(6), 1085–1096.

III

Management of the Disease Process

9

The Immune System and Its Role in Multiple Sclerosis

OBJECTIVES

Upon completion of this chapter, the learner will be able to:

- *Cite normal immune system activity*
- *Discuss abnormal immunology involved in multiple sclerosis (MS)*
- *Describe the rationale for immunomodulating MS treatments*

- The immune system protects people from pathogens such as:
  A. Bacteria
  B. Viruses
  C. Parasites
  D. Fungi

- The immune system protects through the mechanisms of:
  A. Innate immunity
  B. Adaptive immunity

- The immune system is a complex interactive network of organs, tissues, cells, cell products, and biochemical mediators.

■ . Likely underlying the disease is an impairment of immune tolerance to central nervous system (CNS) tissue that ultimately leads to plaque formation.

■ Damage to the axons and axonal loss occur early in the disease, often long before the appearance of clinical symptoms.

■ The immune system is composed of the following:

A. Innate immunity

   1. Immunity to certain pathogens; this is common to all healthy individuals

   2. Does not require prior exposure to the pathogen

   3. Immediate destruction of some pathogens by phagocytic cells such as macrophages and neutrophils

B. Adaptive immunity

   1. Requires exposure to pathogen to stimulate immune system response

   2. Cellular immunity

      a. Cytotoxic T cells (CD8)

      b. T_H cells (CD4)

   3. Humoral immunity

      a. B lymphocytes

      b. Antibodies

C. Cells of the immune system begin life in the bone marrow as stem cells.

D. T cells are differentiated in the thymus.

E. B cells are differentiated in the bone marrow.

F. These cells are activated in the lymphoid tissues, where they are presented with antigen.

G. B cells recognize an antigen that is present outside of cells.

H. T cells detect antigens processed inside host cells and presented on the cell surface.

I. Both B and T cells must receive an additional signal in order to be activated.

■ Humoral immunity

A. Antibodies produced by B cells

B. Antibodies work through a variety of mechanisms, including the following:

   1. Neutralization—binding to pathogens and blocking the path to body cells

2. Opsonization—enabling phagocytic cells to recognize pathogens by coating the pathogen
3. Complement activation

■ Cellular immunity is produced by
A. T lymphocytes each having cell surface receptors:
1. Distinct from lymphocyte to lymphocyte.
2. This enables lymphocytes to recognize a wide variety of antigens.
B. Once a T cell is activated by antigen presentation:
1. It proliferates in a process known as *clonal expansion*.
2. Antigen-specific lymphocytes undergo apoptosis once the antigen is removed.
3. Some antigen-specific lymphocytes persist: memory T cells.
4. The cells that present antigen to T cells are antigen-presenting cells:
   a. Dendritic cells
   b. Macrophages
5. These cells display antigen protein particles on speciaized cell surface molecules known as major histocompatibility complexes (MHCs).
6. Two classes of MHC molecules exist:
   a. MHC I
   b. MHC II
7. MHC I are recognized by cytotoxic T cells (CD8).
8. MHC II are expressed on the surface of macrophages or B cells and are recognized by T_H1 or T_H2 cells (CD4).
9. CD4 cell cytokine production
   a. T_H1 cells activate macrophages and produce
      I. Interferon-gamma (IFN-γ)
      II. TNF-α
      III. TNF-β
      IV. IL-2
   b. T_H2 cells activate B cells and produce
      I. IL-4
      II. IL-5
      III. IL-10
      IV. TGF-β

■ Inappropriate immune response includes

A. Allergy

B. Autoimmune disease

■ Allergy is the result of a specific immunoglobulin E (IgE) antibody to an innocuous antigen.

■ In autoimmune illness

A. T cells that recognize self-antigen are normally deleted.

B. The regulatory mechanisms that keep these cells in check are not working properly.

C. Without regulation, autoreactive T cells can proliferate.

D. Molecular mimicry occurs

1. Self-protein is structurally similar to non–self-antigen.

2. T cells can recognize self-antigens if they are sufficiently similar to the non–self-antigen.

■ In multiple sclerosis (MS)

A. T_H cells are stimulated in the periphery by presentation with antigen (i.e., a virus particle). These naive T cells are stimulated to be inflammatory (T_H1) or anti-inflammatory (T_H2). In MS inflammation, activation of T_H1 occurs. In MS, these T_H cells include cells that react to CNS tissue such as myelin basic protein.

B. Once activated, they proliferate and release cytokines and metalloproteinases that break down the extracellular matrix of the blood–brain barrier (BBB).

C. Once in the CNS, T_H1 cells are presented with myelin protein that is similar to the antigen presented in the periphery.

D. The T_H1 cells are thus reactivated.

E. Once reactivated, they release damaging cytokines, such as IFN-γ, TNF-α, TNF-β, and IL-2, and recruit other inflammatory cells to the area.

■ New areas of research in experimental autoimmune encephalomyelitis (the experimental model of MS) and human MS have identified previously unknown contributions to disease pathogenesis, including interleukin-17-producing T helper 17 cells, B cells, CD8⁺ T cells, and both CD4⁺ and CD8⁺ T-regulatory cells.

■ Research into the respective mechanisms of action of these cells has identified novel therapeutic targets to combat this devastating disease.

■ Disease-modifying treatments include the following:
A. Selective immunomodulation
   1. Glatiramer acetate (Copaxone)
   2. Dimethyl fumarate (Tecfidera)
B. Nonspecific immunomodulation
   1. IFNβ-1a (Avonex, Plegridy, Rebif)
   2. IFNβ-1b (Betaseron, Extavia)
C. Selective adhesion molecule inhibitor
   1. Natalizumab (Tysabri)
D. Sphingosine 1-phosphate receptor modulator
   1. Fingolimod (Gilenya)
E. Immunosuppression
   1. Mitoxantrone (Novantrone)
   2. Alemtuzumab (Lemtrada)
   3. Teriflunomide (Aubagio)

■ Immunomodulating and immunosuppressive agents have an effect on some aspect of the immune response; with some agents, the effect is general, with others more specific.
A. IFN-β thought to:
   1. Inhibit T cell proliferation
   2. Inhibit synthesis of inflammatory cytokines (IFN-γ, TNF-α)
   3. Downregulate expression of MHC class II molecules induced by IFN-γ
   4. Reduce antigen presentation to T cells
   5. Downregulate adhesion molecules and promote BBB integrity
   6. Stimulate production of IL-10, a regulatory cytokine
B. Glatiramer acetate thought to:
   1. Induce suppressor T cells
   2. Be structurally similar to myelin basic protein. When glatiramer acetate (GA) induced T cells are presented to myelin basic protein (MBP) in the CNS, it is felt that they are stimulated to proliferate and release cytokines (TGF-β, IL-4, IL-10).
C. Mitoxantrone thought to:
   1. Produce a broad spectrum of immunosuppression with some B-cell suppression.

D. Cyclophosphamide thought to:

1. Produce broad-spectrum immunosuppressant.

E. Imuran thought to:

1. Produce broad-spectrum immunosuppressant with B-cell suppression.

F. Methotrexate used off label:

1. As an immunosuppressant used in other autoimmune diseases and has been used in MS for a number of years.

G. Natalizumab

1. The U.S. Food and Drug Administration (USFDA) approved in 2004; withdrawn from the market in 2005; reentered the market in 2006 with safety monitoring in North America.

2. Blocks adhesion molecules on the surface of T cells, thus preventing adhesion to the BBB and migration into the CNS.

H. Fingolimod (FTY7320)

1. Approved by the FDA in 2010.

2. A synthetic analog of sphingosie-1-phosphate and is an oral medication.

3. Acts by high-level binding blocking signals necessary for migration of T cells from lymphoid tissue and the thymus, thus preventing them from migrating into the CNS.

I. Teriflunomide

1. Oral immunomodulator with anti-inflammatory activity dehydrogenase (DHO-DH).

2. DHO-DH is the fourth enzyme and rate-limiting step in the de novo synthesis pathway of pyrimidines (crucial for replicating DNA and RNA).

3. It inhibits rapidly dividing cell populations and is nonspecific to T cell.

J. Dimethyl fumarate

1. Oral dimethyl fumarate (DMF) activates the nuclear factor (erythroid-derived 2)-like 2 (Nrf2) transcriptional pathway.

2. Defends against oxidative stress-induced neuronal death.

3. Protects the BBB.

4. Supports maintenance of myelin integrity in the CNS.

5. Experimental evidence suggests that DMF may provide anti-inflammatory and cytoprotective effects in the treatment of MS.

6. Induces anti-inflammatory T_H2 cytokines.

7. Shown to increase IL-10 and decrease TNF-α and IL-6.

8. Induces apoptosis in activated T cells.

9. Induces expression of phase 2 detoxification enzymes in astroglial and microglial cells.

10. Reduces the expression of adhesion molecules.

K. Alemtuzumab

1. Humanized monoclonal antibody directed at CD52 (an antigen found on T lymphocytes, B lymphocytes, and monocytes).

2. Cytolytic effect—reduces circulating:

a. T cells

b. B cells

c. Natural killer cells

3. Originally approved in the United States and European Union in 2001 and approved for B-CLL (B-cell chronic lymphocytic leukemia).

4. Approved for MS in Canada and EU in 2014; US in 2015.

■ Treating MS early with disease-modifying drugs is important because:

A. Relapses and impairment have been shown to parallel MRI burden of disease.

B. Axonal damage occurs early and may cause permanent neurologic dysfunction.

C. Number of MRI lesions may be predictive of future disability.

D. Preventing development of lesions may delay progression of disability.

E. Preventing early relapses may delay long-term disability.

RESOURCES

Abbas, A., & Lichtman, A. (2006). *Basic immunology: Functions and disorders of the immune system* (2nd ed.). Philadelphia, PA: Saunders Elsevier.

Antel, J. P., & Bar-Or, A. (2003). Do myelin-directed antibodies predict multiple sclerosis? *New England Journal of Medicine, 349,* 107–109.

Chaplin, D. D. (2003). Overview of the immune response. *Journal of Allergy and Clinical Immunology, 111*(Suppl. 2), S442–S459.

Fox, E. J., Lisak, R. P., & Connor, C. S. (Eds.). (2009). *Clinician's primer on multiple sclerosis: Immunology and the basic mechanisms of action of pharmacological and therapeutic agents.* Denver, CO: Consensus Medical Education Communications and Medical Education Resources.

Goverman, J. (2009). Autoimmune T cell responses: I: The central nervous system. *Nature Reviews Immunology, 9,* 393–407.

Halper, J. (2007). The nature of multiple sclerosis. In J. Halper (Ed.), *Advanced concepts in multiple sclerosis nursing care* (pp. 1–26). New York, NY: Demos Medical.

Halper, J., & Holland, N. J. (2011). An overview of multiple sclerosis. In J. Halper & N. J. Holland (Eds.), *Comprehensive nursing care in multiple sclerosis* (2nd ed., pp. 1–16). New York, NY: Springer Publishing Company.

Kasper, L. H., & Shomaker, J. (2010). Multiple sclerosis immunology: The healthy immune system vs. the MS immune system. *Neurology, 74*(Suppl. 1), S2–S8.

Magliozzi, R., Howell, O., Vora, A., Serafni, B., Nicholas, R., Puopolo, M., . . . Aloisi, F. (2007). Meningeal B-cell follicles in secondary progressive multiple sclerosis associate with early onset of disease and severe cortical pathology. *Brain, 130,* 1089–1104.

McFarland, H. F., & Martin, R. (2007). Multiple sclerosis: A complicated picture of autoimmunity. *Nature Immunology, 8*(9), 913–919.

Paty, D. W., & Ebers, G. C. (1998). *Multiple sclerosis.* Philadelphia, PA: F.A. Davis.

Porter, B., Costello, K., Halper, J., Harris, C., & Perrin Ross, A. (2004). *Topics in multiple sclerosis: An immunological perspective.* Somerville, NJ: The Whitaker-McFarlin MS Colloquium, Embryon.

Traugott, U. (2001). Evidence for immunopathogenesis. In S. D. Cook (Ed.), *Handbook of multiple sclerosis* (3rd ed., pp. 163–192). New York, NY: Marcel Dekker.

Wekerle, H., & Hehlfeld, R. (2003). Molecular mimicry in multiple sclerosis. *New England Journal of Medicine, 349,* 185–186.

Yong, W. (2002). Differential mechanisms of action of interferon β and glatiramer acetate in MS. *Neurology, 59,* 802–808.

10

Multiple Sclerosis: Managing the Disease

OBJECTIVES

Upon completion of this chapter, the learner will be able to:

■ Discuss relapse management in multiple sclerosis (MS)
■ Describe U.S. Food and Drug Administration–approved disease modification in relapsing forms of MS
■ List treatment patterns using off-label therapies, and describe strategies to promote adherence to complex protocols

■ Relapse management
   A. A *relapse* is the appearance of a new symptom or the reappearance of a previous symptom of multiple sclerosis (MS) after the initial attack. A relapse cannot be related to an intercurrent infection or any other environmental factors and must last more than 24 hours.
   B. In clinical practice, relapses are usually managed with high-dose intravenous or oral corticosteroids for a limited amount of time:
      1. Methylprednisolone
      2. Prednisone

3. Dexamethasone

4. Adrenocorticotropic hormone (ACTH)

5. Medrol

C. No proof of benefit on relapse rates and progression. Corticosteroids are known to shorten the duration of the relapse, but may not affect the overall disease course. Chronic steroids are not recommended because of lack of evidence of benefit and side effects (hematologic effects, bone loss, and increased susceptibility to infection).

D. Minimal evidence on optimal dose or regimen.

E. Protocols vary from country to country.

■ Immunosuppressant therapies

A. Azathioprine (oral) not approved for MS

1. Was used a great deal in the 1970s before injectable medications were approved

2. Recent evidence suggests slight effect on disease activity when compared with an interferon product

3. Recommendation not to exceed 600 mg daily in view of possible risk of malignancy

B. Cyclophosphamide (intravenous or oral) not approved for MS

1. Conflicting studies

2. High adverse-effect profile

3. Many varying protocols

4. May be used for "rescue therapy"

5. There are dose-related toxicities

C. Methotrexate (oral) not approved for MS

1. Paucity of evidence of effectiveness, including MRI

2. Weekly low dose may help delay progression in progressive MS

3. Research demonstrates modest effect on upper-extremity function

4. Must be taken daily with folic acid

5. Anecdotal reports of use of combination therapy

D. Mitoxantrone (intravenous)

1. Studied widely in Europe

2. Approved by the U.S. Food and Drug Administration for worsening forms of relapsing MS

3. Used in aggressive, relapsing MS and in patients with inadequate response to disease-modifying agents (DMAs)

4. Has lifetime maximal dose

    5. Potential for cardiotoxicity

    6. Documented risk for leukemia

E. Intravenous immunoglobulin not approved for MS

    1. Obtained from blood of healthy human donors

    2. Several studies with conflicting results

    3. Used in Devic syndrome (neuromyelitis optica spectrum disorder)

    4. Well tolerated

    5. Very costly

■ Approved disease-modifying therapies (DMTs)

A. Therapies becoming available worldwide

B. Reimbursement for costs varies widely throughout states in the United States and provinces of Canada

C. In most countries, available for relapsing MS

D. Therapy initiation and ongoing adherence require nursing services (documented in research)

E. Available therapies

    1. Interferon-β (1b, 1a intramuscular and subcutaneous)

    2. Glatiramer acetate

    3. Natalizumab

    4. Fingolimod

    5. Teriflunomide

    6. Dimethyl fumarate

    7. Alemtuzumab

F. Interferon-β 1b (Betaseron or Betaferon or Extavia)

    1. 8 MIU subcutaneously every other day

    2. Requires reconstitution

    3. Diluent available in prefilled syringe

    4. Autoinjector for injection

    5. Benefit in relapse rates and MRI

    6. Preliminary data on cognition and depression

    7. In secondary-progressive MS, North American study was not statistically significant; in Europe, the results were positive

    8. Delayed onset of clinically definite MS by 1 year in BENEFIT trial

    9. Approved for clinically isolated syndrome (CIS) patients

    10. No clinical benefit found by studies comparing interferon-β to glatiramer acetate, although MRI benefit seen (BECOME and BEYOND studies)

11. Side-effect profile:
    a. Flu-like syndrome
    b. Skin reactions and rare necrosis
    c. Menstrual changes, abortifacient potential
    d. Reports of depression (refuted in 2002, Feinstein, O'Connor, & Feinstein)
    e. Neutralizing antibodies 38%
    f. Leukopenia
    g. Elevated liver enzymes
    h. Thrombocytopenia
12. Side-effect management includes patient and family education in dose titration, timing of injections, nonsteroidal anti-inflammatory drugs (NSAIDs), site rotation, management of depression
13. Regular blood work important more frequently initially and at regular intervals thereafter
G. Interferon-β 1a (Avonex)
    1. 30 mcg (6 MIU) intramuscular injection once weekly—prefilled syringe
    2. Slows progression measured by Expanded Disability Status Scale (EDSS) in relapsing MS
    3. Reduces relapses by 18%
    4. Delays onset of Certification of Disability Management Specialists (CDMS) by 1 year (monosymptomatic trial-CHAMPS); approved for CIS
    5. No clear benefit in secondary-progressive MS
    6. Benefit in brain atrophy reported
    7. Side effects include:
       a. Flu-like syndrome
       b. Cautious use with seizures or depression
       c. Abortifacient potential
       d. Neutralizing antibodies
       e. Elevated liver enzymes
    8. Side-effect management includes patient and family education, timing of injections, NSAIDs, site rotation, and management of depression
H. Interferon-β 1a (Rebif)
    1. Two doses (22 and 44 mcg) three times weekly subcutaneously
    2. Prefilled syringes with autoinjector (Rebiject)

3. Dose-dependent decrease in relapse and MRI disease burden
4. Delayed onset of clinically definite MS by 9 months (ETOMS study)
5. Side effects include:
    a. Flu-like syndrome
    b. Site reactions and rare necrosis
    c. Menstrual irregularities
    d. Leukopenia, elevated liver enzymes, and thrombocytopenia
    e. Neutralizing antibodies
    f. Possible depression, although this was refuted in a recent study
6. Side-effect management includes patient and family education in dose titration, timing of injections, NSAIDs, site rotation, and management of depression

I. Glatiramer acetate (Copaxone; combination of four amino acids)
1. 20 mg subcutaneously daily
2. In prefilled syringe with autoinjector
3. Sustained benefit in reduction of relapse rate
4. Significant reduction of MRI lesion number and volume
5. No benefit for primary progressive MS (PROMISE trial)
6. No statistical significance in oral form (CORAL trial)
7. PreCISE trial demonstrated benefit in CIS; medication approved for early disease
8. Side effects include:
    a. Injection site reaction, hives, and pain
    b. Rare systemic reaction (chest pain, dyspnea, and anxiety— postinjection reaction)
    c. Arthralgia and nausea

J. Common problems with disease modifying therapies (DMTs)
1. Spasticity
    a. Can be seen in patients with greater disability
    b. Commonly seen with interferon therapy
    c. May occur on initiation of therapy or prior to treatment
    d. Differential diagnosis between interferon-induced spasticity and spasticity associated with relapse or infection is necessary
    e. Assess for other contributing factors
    f. Administer antispasticity medications
    g. Consider dose adjustment of interferons until problem is managed

2. Laboratory abnormalities

   a. No known significant abnormalities with glatiramer acetate

   b. In interferon therapy, the most common abnormalities are leukopenia, neutropenia, and raised liver aminotransferase values (e.g., serum glutamic oxaloacetic and serum glutamic pyruvic transaminase)

3. Managing laboratory abnormalities

   a. Monitor laboratory values regularly following initiation of treatment, and yearly thereafter

   b. Inform physician of abnormal values

   c. Consider dose adjustment and/or discontinuation of treatment if abnormalities persist

4. Depression

   a. Common in MS

   b. Conflicting data about relationship to interferon therapy

   c. Expert opinion is to treat depression before starting DMTs

K. Natalizumab (intravenous)

   1. Monoclonal antibody designed to interfere with movement of potentially damaging immune cells across the blood–brain barrier.

   2. Showed significant reduction of annual relapse rate (68% reduction), sustained progression and reduction in both new T2 lesions (83%) and gadolinium-enhancing MRI lesions (92%).

   3. Side effects include headache, fatigue, urinary tract infections, joint pain, and abdominal discomfort.

   4. Voluntarily withdrawn from market because of serious adverse events of progressive multifocal leukoencephalopathy (PML) after approval in 2004; withdrawn in 2005; rereleased in 2006 with safety monitoring in place in North America. PML is a serious, potentially disabling, or fatal brain infection caused by the John Cunningham (JC) virus. The JC virus is a common virus that is harmless in most people, but can cause PML in a small number of people treated with certain types of MS drug therapies, and is thought to be due to an unusual immune response to the JC virus.

   5. Given every 4 weeks by infusion.

   6. Patients should be screened for signs and symptoms of premenstrual syndrome (PMS; altered mental status, altered function, and depression) before each infusion, along with monitoring for systemic infection.

L. Fingolimod (Gilenya)

   1. Oral immunomodulator/immunosuppressant taken once daily

2. Sequesters mainly T lymphocytes in lymph nodes, which is reversed when drug is discontinued

3. Showed reduction in relapse rate, MRI indicators of disease activity, and impact on brain atrophy

4. Recommended screening prior to initiation of therapy includes ophthalmology, cardiology, and dermatology if there is a family history of skin malignancies

5. Patients must be tested for rubella antibodies; if negative, must have immunization and wait 2 months to start the medication

6. Bradycardia occurs with the first dose; therefore, a 6-hour monitoring period is in the labeling of the medication

7. Other side effects include headache, hypertension, breathlessness, decreased resistance to infection, visual blurring, and ocular pain (macular edema must be ruled out)

8. There have been several occurrences of PML

9. Routine follow-up blood work that includes complete blood count (CBC), creatinine, alkaline phosphatase, bilirubin, TSH, follow-up eye exams, and pulmonary function tests where appropriate

M. Teriflunomide

1. Active metabolite of leflunomide, FDA-approved for rheumatoid arthritis

2. An oral immunomodulator with anti-inflammatory activity inhibits pyrimidine synthesis by binding to the enzyme dihydro-orotate dehydrogenase

3. Inhibits rapidly dividing cell populations and is nonspecific to T cells

4. Teriflunomide 14 mg taken once daily showed impact on relapse rate and MRI indicators of disease activity

5. Side effects include elevated liver enzymes, gastrointestinal disturbance, lymphopenia, and hair thinning

6. Teratogenic for men and women

7. Monthly CBC and liver function tests (LFTs) for at least 6 months recommended

8. Slow excretion of this medication, not dialyzable, and present in blood levels for 8 to 24 months after discontinuation

9. Accelerated elimination is available with cholestyramine 8 g, po q8 hours × 11 days or activated charcoal 50 g po q12 hours × 11 days

N. Dimethyl fumarate (DMF)

1. First approved to treat psoriasis in the form of Fumarate

2. In MS, acts as immunomodulator, and experimental evidence suggests that DMF may provide anti-inflammatory and cyto-protective effects in the treatment of MS

3. Oral medication given in doses of 240 mg twice daily as tolerated in DEFINE and CONFIRM trial

4. Showed impact on relapses and MRI indicators of disease activity

5. Side effects include generalized flushing and GI disturbances, including diarrhea and intestinal cramping and bloating

6. There have been several occurrences of PML

7. Regular blood work includes CBC, creatinine, alkaline phosphatase, bilirubin, TSH, and urinalysis for presence of protein

O. Alemtuzumab

1. Alemtuzumab, a humanized monoclonal antibody, has shown efficacy for relapsing–remitting multiple sclerosis in phase 2 and phase 3 trials. Compared with subcutaneous interferon β-1a, alemtuzumab significantly reduced the risk for accumulation of disability and the rate of relapse, and improved mean disability level from baseline.

2. Side effects include infusion-associated reactions, infections of predominantly mild-to-moderate severity, and autoimmune adverse events (principally, thyroid disorders and immune thrombocytopenia).

3. Pivotal trials showed reduction of annual relapse rate of 55% and decreased worsening of progression as compared with beta interferon 1a by subcutaneous injection.

4. Alemtuzumab 12 mg intravenous infusion is given once a day for 5 days, followed 1 year later by 12 mg intravenous infusion once a day for 3 days.

5. Patients require prescreening immunizations and blood work as well as regular postinfusion blood monitoring including CBC, creatinine, alkaline phosphatase, bilirubin, and thyroid stimulating hormone (TSH)—monthly for 48 months following last infusion.

■ Emerging therapies and therapies under review

A. Laquinimod—in investigation

1. Oral medication that appears to modulate cytokine balance in favor of T_H2/T_H3 cytokines (anti-inflammatory)

2. ALLEGRO study showed reduction in relapse rate and EDSS progression

3. BRAVO trial compares laquinimod with placebo and interferon-β 1a

4. CONCERTO, a follow-up phase III study, scheduled for completion in 2018, will examine disability progression in participants treated with placebo, 0.6 mg laquinimod, or 1.2 mg laquinimod

5. Main adverse effect appears to be self-limited, dose-dependent increase in liver enzymes

B. Ocrelizumab (submitted to FDA for approval)

1. An anti-CD 20 monoclonal antibody that lyses circulating B cells.

2. Both the OPERA I and II studies in relapsing–remitting MS and the ORATORIO trial in primary progressive MS met primary end points.

3. The OPERA studies suggested ocrelizumab may be a highly effective agent in relapsing–remitting MS, but without the serious adverse effects seen with other, similarly potent agents.

4. ORATORIO trial is the first phase 3 study to show a slowing of disability progression in primary progressive MS.

5. Medication is well tolerated.

C. Autologous hematopoietic stem cell transplantation

1. Bone marrow transplantation, with a patient's own bone marrow stem cells, is an aggressive and risky treatment that is currently reserved for a small subgroup of patients with early aggressive MS that does not respond to other therapies.

2. Results of trials have shown that most patients had no further relapses and no new lesions visible by MRI for 2 years following the treatment, but the progressive process does continue.

3. Most cells of the immune system were restored following the treatment, including the types of T cells that can react to myelin in the brain (autoreactive T cells). Another type of cell, known as T_H17, remained reduced in number following the procedure, and T_H17 immune function did not return to normal.

4. T_H17 cells are known to be involved in crossing the blood–brain barrier and may assist other immune cells such as inflammatory T_H1 cells and autoreactive T cells to enter the brain.

5. Research is ongoing and is being used as rescue therapy in some centers throughout the world.

■ Initiation of therapy: Sustaining adherence

A. Neurologists, advanced practice nurses, physician assistants, and primary care physicians may be involved in treatment decisions. Regardless of who makes the decision, it is imperative that the nurse educate the patient and family on the following:

1. All available treatments

2. Efficacy and side effects

3. Self-care activities

4. The importance of adherence

■ The psychoeducational approach

A. Requires that the patient and family become actively involved in goal setting, realistic expectations, and the process itself

B. Patient and family education requirements

1. Information is provided in a clear and concise manner.

2. A relaxed and nondistracting learning environment is available.

3. A variety of educational tools are used.

4. Reinforcement is provided regularly.

5. Education should not be initiated immediately after diagnosis.

6. Hope can be instilled along with realistic expectations.

7. Patients must be motivated to learn; if they are not ready, education should be delayed.

8. Educational strategies must take into account patient's age, cultural and educational background, and previous experience with the health care system.

9. Outcomes of education; patients should be able to

a. Describe rationale of therapy

b. Correctly reconstitute and administer medication

c. Manage side effects

d. Identify and use resources to obtain further information

10. Promoting adherence

a. Establishment of a trusting relationship

b. Consistent and clear education

c. Advocacy for access to treatment

d. Reinforcement by the multidisciplinary team during ongoing patient and family contact

RESOURCES

Atkins, L., & Freedman, M. (2013). Hematopoetic stem cell therapy for multiple sclerosis: Top 10 lessons learned. *Neurotherapeutics, 10*(1), 68–76.

Bourdette, D., Yadav, V., & Shinto, L. (2004). Multiple sclerosis. In B. S. Oken (Ed.), *Complementary therapies in neurology: An evidence-based approach* (pp. 291–302). New York, NY: Parthenon.

Bowling, A. C. (2006). *Alternative medicine and multiple sclerosis* (2nd ed.). New York, NY: Demos Medical Publishing.

Burks, J., & Johnson, K. P. (Eds). (2000). *Multiple sclerosis: Diagnosis, medical management, rehabilitation*. New York, NY: Demos Medical Publishing.

Cassetta, I., Iuliano, G., & Filippini, G. (2009). Azathioprine for multiple sclerosis. *Journal of Neurology, Neurosurgery, and Psychiatry, 80*(2), 131–132.

Cohen, B. A., & Rieckmann, P. (2007). Emerging oral therapies for multiple sclerosis. *International Journal of Clinical Practice, 61*, 1922–1930.

Cohen, J. A. (2009). Emerging therapies for relapsing multiple sclerosis. *Archives of Neurology, 66*, 1922–1930.

Cohen, J. A., Coles, A. J., Arnold, D. L., Confavreux, C., Fox, E. J., Hartung, H. P., . . . Compston, D. A.; for the CARE-MS I Investigators. (2012). Alemtuzumab versus interferon beta 1a as first-line treatment for patients with relapsing-remitting multiple sclerosis: A randomised controlled phase 3 trial. *Lancet, 380*(9856), 1819–1828.

Comi, G., O'Connor, P., Montalban, X., Antel, J., Radue, E., Karlsson G., . . . Kappos, L.; FTY720D2201 Study Group. (2010). Phase II study of oral fingolimod (FTY720) in multiple sclerosis: 3-year results. *Multiple Sclerosis, 16*(2), 197–207.

Costello, K., & Halper, J. (2010a). *Multiple sclerosis: Key issues in nursing management: Adherence, cognition, quality of life*. New York, NY: Bioscience.

Costello, K., & Halper, J. (2010b). *Advanced practice nursing in multiple sclerosis: Advanced skills, advancing responsibilities.* Washington, DC: EME.

Costello, K., Halper, J., Morgante, L., & Namey, M. D. (2005). *Case management in multiple sclerosis*. Teaneck, NJ: International Organization of MS Nurses.

Costello, K., Kennedy, P., & Scanzillo, J. (2008). Recognizing nonadherence in patients with multiple sclerosis and maintaining treatment adherence in the long term. *Medscape Journal of Medicine, 10*, 225.

Fraser, C., Hadjimichael, O., & Vollmer, T. (2001). Predictors of adherence to copaxone therapy in individuals with relapsing-remitting multiple sclerosis. *Journal of Neuroscience Nursing, 33*, 231–239.

Fraser, C., Hadjimichael, O., & Vollmer, T. (2003). Predictors of adherence to glatiramer acetate therapy in individuals with self-reported progressive forms of multiple sclerosis. *Journal of Neuroscience Nursing, 35*, 163–170.

Feinstein A., O'Connor P., & Feinstein K. (2002). Multiple sclerosis, interferon beta-1b and depression: A prospective investigation. *Journal of Neurology, 249*(7):815–820.

Giovannoni, G., Comi, G., Cook, S., Rammohan, K., Rieckmann, P., Sørensen, P. S., . . . Greenberg S. J.; for the CLARITY Study Group (2010). A-placebo-controlled trial of oral cladribine for relapsing multiple sclerosis. *New England Journal of Medicine, 362,* 416–426.

Gold, R. (2011). Oral therapies for multiple sclerosis: A review of agents in phase III development or recently approved. *CNS Drugs, 25,* 37–52.

Gold, R., Kappos, L., Bar-Or, D., Arnold, D., Giovannoni, G., Selmaj, K., . . . Dawson, K. (2011). Clinical efficacy of BG-12, an oral therapy, in relapsing-remitting multiple sclerosis. Data from the phase 3 DEFINE trial [Abstract 95]. *Multiple Sclerosis, 17*(Suppl. 10), S34.

Goodin, D. S., Frohman, E. M., Garmany, G. P., Jr., Halper, J., Likosky, W. H., Lublin, F. D., . . . van den Noort, S.; Therapeutics and Technology Assessment Subcommittee of the American Academy of Neurology and the MS Council for Clinical Practice Guidelines. (2002). Disease modifying therapies in multiple sclerosis: Report of the Therapeutics and Technology Assessment Subcommittee of the American Academy of Neurology and the MS Council for Clinical Practice Guidelines. *Neurology, 58*(2), 169–177.

Halper, J. (2007). The nature of multiple sclerosis. In J. Halper (Ed.), *Advanced concepts in multiple sclerosis nursing care* (pp. 1–26). New York, NY: Demos Medical.

Halper, J., & Holland, N. J. (2011). An overview of multiple sclerosis. In J. Halper & N. J. Holland (Eds.), *Comprehensive nursing care in multiple sclerosis* (pp. 1–16). New York, NY: Springer Publishing Company.

Harris, C., & Halper, J. (2008). *Best practices in nursing care: Disease management, pharmacological treatment, nursing research.* New York, NY: Bioscience.

Kamin, S. S. (2011, Spring). New and emerging therapies in multiple sclerosis: The team approach to decision making. *International Journal of MS Care, 13*(Suppl. 1), 1–24.

Kappos, L., Antel, J., Comi, G., Montalban, X., O'Connor, P., Polman C., . . . Radue, E.; FTY720 D2201 Study Group. (2006). Oral fingolimod (FTY720) for relapsing multiple sclerosis. *New England Journal of Medicine, 55*(11), 1124–1140.

Kappos, L., Radue, E. W., O'Connor, P., Polman, C., Hohlfeld, R., Calabresi, P., . . . Burtin P.; FREEDOMS Study Group.(2010). A placebo-controlled trial of oral fingolimod in relapsing multiple sclerosis. *New England Journal of Medicine, 362*(5), 387–401.

McDonald, I. W., & Noseworthy, J. H. (Eds.). (2003). *Blue books of practical neurology: Multiple sclerosis 2.* New York, NY: Elsevier Science.

O'Connor, P., Wolinsky, J. S., Confavreux, C., Comi, G., Kappos, L., Olsson, T. P., . . . Freedman, M. S.; TEMSO Trial Group. (2011). Randomized trial of oral teriflunomide for relapsing multiple sclerosis. *New England Journal of Medicine, 365*(14), 1293–1303.

Patti, F. (2010). Optimizing the benefit of multiple sclerosis therapy: The importance of treatment adherence. *Patient Preference and Adherence, 4,* 1–9.

Radaelli, M., Merlini, A., Greco, R., Sangalli, F., Giancarlo, C., Fabio C., & Martino, M. (2014). Autologous bone marrow transplantation for the treatment of multiple sclerosis. *Current Neurology and Neuroscience Reports, 14*(478), 7–13.

Twork, S., Nippert, I., Scherer, P., Haas, J., Pohlau, D., & Kugler, J. (2007). Immunomodulating drugs in multiple sclerosis: Compliance, satisfaction and adverse effects evaluation in a German multiple sclerosis population. *Current Medical Research and Opinion, 23,* 1209–1215.

Van den Noort, S., & Holland, N. J. (Eds.). (1999). *Multiple sclerosis in clinical practice.* New York, NY: Demos Medical.

IV

Functional Alterations: Physical Domains

11

The Symptom Chain in Multiple Sclerosis

OBJECTIVES

Upon completion of this chapter, the learner will be able to:

- Describe the most common symptoms of multiple sclerosis (MS)
- Cite effective management strategies for MS symptoms
- Discuss the nurse's role in symptomatic management

- Multiple sclerosis (MS) is a complex and dynamic disease.
  A. In addition to different disease courses, symptoms can be disabling if not managed adequately.
  B. Signs and symptoms vary from person to person or within the individual from time to time or consistently.
  C. Fluctuation may be based on the following circumstances:
    1. Environmental factors such as heat or humidity
    2. Metabolic factors such as underlying infection
    3. The disease itself during relapses and/or a worsening course
  D. Many symptoms have a cascade effect on functioning.
  E. Careful management can improve quality of life.

    F. Inadequately controlled symptomatic problems can be major challenges for the patient and the nursing professional.

    G. There is a need for ongoing vigilance and assessment.

    H. Patient and family education are vital throughout a lifetime with MS to assist the patient and family to differentiate between symptomatic problems, relapses, and worsening disease.

    I. It is essential to support the patient's safety and maximal functional status.

- The key to management is knowledge and skills.

    A. Symptoms must be recognized, understood, and discussed with the health care team by the patient and family.

    B. Management should be individualized and flexible in light of the dynamic nature of MS.

    C. Patient and professional collaboration are essential for successful symptomatic management.

    D. Symptom control may consist of both pharmacologic and non-pharmacologic strategies.

- Common symptoms of MS (Table 11.1)

    A. Fatigue

    B. Depression

    C. Focal muscle weakness

    D. Visual changes

    E. Bowel, bladder, and sexual dysfunction

    F. Gait problems, spasticity

    G. Paresthesias

    H. Neuropathic pain (see Chapter 16)

- Less common symptoms of MS

    A. Dysarthria, scanning speech, and dysphagia

    B. Lhermitte's sign

    C. Ataxia

    D. Vertigo

    E. Cognitive dysfunction

    F. Tremor, incoordination

- Rare symptoms of MS

    A. Decreased hearing

    B. Convulsions

Table 11.1 Pharmacologic Information

MS symptom	Generic name	Brand name	Usual dosage
MS relapse	Adrenocortico-tropic hormone (ACTH)	ACTHAR gel	80–100 U/d × 2 wk IM, IV
	Methylpredniso-lone	Solu-Medrol	1 g IV × 3–5 d
	Dexamethasone	Decadron	160–180 mg/d × 3–5 d (po) or 30 mg tapered × 10 d (po)
	Prednisone	Deltasone	Given initially in high doses and tapered per prescriber preference (po)
MS fatigue	Modafinil	Provigil	100–200 mg/d (po)
	Armodafinil	Nuvigil	150 or 250 mg/d (po)
	Methylphenidate	Ritalin	This medication can be taken either twice daily or three times daily per the precriber's instructions
	Dextroamphet-mine	Dexedrine	5–60 mg tid (po)
	Amantidine	Symmetrel	100 mg bid or tid (po)
Depression	Fluoxetine	Prozac	20–80 mg/d (po)
	Paroxetine	Paxil/Paxil CR	20–50 mg/ 25–62.5 mg (po)
	Sertraline	Zoloft	100–200 mg/d (po)
	Citalopram	Celexa	20–60 mg/d (po)
	Escitalopam	Lexapro	10–20 mg/d (po)
	Fluvoxamine	Luvox	100–300 mg/d (po)
	Venlafaxine	Effexor XR	50–375 mg/d (po)
	Duloxetine	Cymbalta	40–60 mg/d (po)
	Amitriptyline	Elavil	100–300 mg/d (po)

(continued)

Table 11.1 Pharmacologic Information *(continued)*

MS symptom	Generic name	Brand name	Usual dosage
Depression	Desipramine	Norpramin	100–300 mg/d (po)
	Imipramine	Tofranil	100–300 mg/d (po)
	Buproprion	Wellbutrin/ XL	75–100 mg/150– 300 mg XL (po)
Urinary dysfunction			
Antimicrobials	Sulfonamide	Sulfamethox- azole and Trimethoprim	SMZ + TMP id × 10–14 d (po)
	Cephalosporin	Keflex	Per prescriber preference po (250–500 mg) or IV
Quinolones	Ciprofloxacin	Cipro	Per prescriber preference
	Levofloxacin	Levaquin	
	Oxfloxacin	Floxin	
	Norfloxacin	Noroxin	
	Gatifloxacin	Tequin	
	Gemifloxacin	Factive	
	Moxifloxacin	Avelox	
Urinary antiseptics	Methenamine	Hiprex	1 g bid (po)
		Mandelamine	500 mg (po)
Urinary urgency/ frequency	Oxybutinin	Ditropan, Ditropan XL	5–30 mg qid/XL 30 mg/d (po)
	Oxybutynin patch	Oxytrol	3.9 mg twice weekly
	Fesoterodine	Toviaz	4 or 8 mg/d (po)
	Tolterodine	Detrol/LA	1–2 mg bid; LA 2–4 mg/d (po)
	Denifenacin	Enablex	7.5–15 mg/d (po)
	Solifenacin	Vesicare	5–10 mg/d (po)
	Trospium	Sanctura	20 mg bid (po)
	Hycoscyamine sulfate	Levsin, Levsinex	0.125–0.25 mg qid/0.375–0.75 mg bid (po)
Urinary hesitancy/ retention	Tamsulosin	Flomax	0.4–0.8 mg after meals
	Terazosin	Hytrin	1–5 mg HS (po)

(continued)

Table 11.1 Pharmacologic Information *(continued)*

MS symptom	Generic name	Brand name	Usual dosage
Bowel dysfunction			
Fecal urgency or incontinence	Imipramine	Tofranil	10, 25, 50 mg/d (po)
	Propantheline	ProBanthine	15 mg bid (po)
Agents for constipation	Docusate	Colace	Over-the-counter products
	Psyllium hydrophilic mucilloid	Metamucil, Konsyl	
	Methylcellulose	Citrucel	
	Glycerine suppository		
	Lactulose	Miralax, Kristalose	
	Polyethylene glycol	Glycolax	By prescription
		GoLytely Colytel, NuLytley	By prescriber
	Fleet enema stimulants	Peri-Colace, Bisacodyl, Senokot, Sagrada	Over-the-counter products
Sexual dysfunction			
Erectile dysfunction	Sildenafil citrate	Viagra	25–100 mg/d (po)
	Tadalafil	Cialis	5–20 mg/d (po)
	Vardenafil	Levitra	2.5–20 mg/d (po)
Spasticity	Baclofen; intrathecal baclofen	Lioresal	20–80 mg/d (po); 25–750 mcg/d (intrathecally)
	Tizanidine	Zanaflex	4–32 mg/d (slow titration)
	Diazepam	Valium	2–10 mg/q or up to qid (po)
	Clonazepam	Klonopin	0.5 mg tid (po)
	Gabapentin	Neurontin	100–900 mg/d (po)

(continued)

Table 11.1 Pharmacologic Information *(continued)*

MS symptom	Generic name	Brand name	Usual dosage
Spasticity	Botulinum toxin A	Botox	IM small muscle groups; approved for upper extremities
Walking problems	Dalfampridine	Ampyra	10 mg bid (po)

bid, twice a day; HS, at bedtime; IM, intramuscular; IV, intravenous; MS, multiple sclerosis; po, orally; qid, four times a day; tid, three times a day.

    C. Tinnitus

    D. Mental disturbance

    E. Paralysis

■ Fatigue

    A. May be directly due to MS (demyelination, immune activity)

    B. Other causes: depression, deconditioning, medications, concomitant medical conditions (thyroid dysfunction, cardiovascular disease), and sleep disturbance

    C. The most common MS symptom

    D. Can be managed using a wide variety of strategies

    E. Evaluation

        1. Assess for impending exacerbation

        2. Screen for infection

        3. Question about environmental factors (heat, humidity)

        4. Ascertain medications, dosages, and time of dosing

        5. Assess sleep habits

        6. Question about other symptoms (pain, spasticity, and bowel or bladder dysfunction)

        7. Assess mood

        8. Evaluate activity level and physical fitness

    F. Management

        1. Instruct in effective energy expenditure

        2. Encourage the appropriate use of assistive devices (scooters, walkers, wheelchairs, and transfer equipment)

3. Encourage the use of air-conditioning and other cooling techniques
4. Encourage the treatment of mood disorders
5. Encourage the initiation of symptom management—pain, spasticity, and bowel and bladder dysfunction
6. Advocate for the treatment of medical conditions causing fatigue
7. Improve sleep hygiene
8. Medications used to manage MS-related fatigue
   a. Central nervous system stimulants (methylphenidate)
   b. Aminopyridine (approved to improve walking in MS)
   c. Amantidine (side effects: headache, dizziness, and rash)
   d. Modafinil (side effects: headache, tachycardia, palpitations, and contraindicated in left ventricular hypertrophy, LMVP)
   e. Selective serotonin reuptake inhibitor (SSRI) antidepressants
   f. Unique antidepressants—bupropion (Wellbutrin; side effect: seizure risk)
9. Initiate appropriate conditioning programs
10. Reassess patient on a regular basis

■ Spasticity

A. Sixty percent of people with MS have corticospinal tract involvement with some degree of spasticity.
B. Accentuation of deep tendon reflexes (DTRs) and clonus occurs, with exaggeration of flexor reflexes.
C. Spasms and stiffness are common in the quadriceps, hamstrings, and gastrocnemius muscles.
D. May be heightened during an exacerbation, with underlying infection, and with noxious stimuli.
E. Physical therapy techniques are designed to:
   1. Avoid secondary complications such as decubitus ulcers
   2. Prevent or treat contractures
   3. Reduce muscle hypertonia by stretching spastic muscles and by application of warm or cold packs
   4. Improve patient's posture
   5. Develop and improve useful automatic movements and thus promote maximal function
   6. Assist the patient to learn more coordinated movements
   7. Supply supportive aids such as walkers, wheelchairs, crutches, orthoses, and special shoes

F. Screening for noxious stimuli will promote prompt treatment and reduction of spasticity

G. Medications for spasticity may be sedating, and excessive doses may result in weakness.

   1. Baclofen

   2. Tizanidine

   3. Clonazepam

   4. Diazepam

H. Intrathecal baclofen

   1. Surgically implanted pump for intrathecal baclofen delivery

      a. Fewer systemic side effects

      b. Expensive

      c. Requires surgery

      d. Reserved for patients in whom other interventions are unsuccessful

■ Tremor, incoordination, and weakness

A. Most difficult problems to modify in MS.

B. Pharmacologic regimens tend to be sedating and have limited benefit.

C. Physical and occupational therapy may provide patient with education and assistive devices, but do not correct the underlying problem.

■ Dysarthria

A. Normal speech consists of five systems working together smoothly and rapidly:

   1. Respiration—using the diaphragm to fill the lungs fully

   2. Phonation—using the vocal cords and airflow

   3. Resonance—raising and lowering the soft palate

   4. Articulation—making quick, precise movements of the lips, tongue, mandible, and soft palate

   5. Prosody—combining all elements for natural flow of speech

B. Speech impairment has long been considered a principal symptom of MS.

C. Three types of dysarthria are associated with MS:

   1. Spastic

   2. Ataxic

   3. Mixed dysarthria

D. In MS, a mixed spastic–ataxic dysarthria is typical.

E. No medications are available for the speech problem itself. Treatment consists of management of spasticity and tremor along with speech and language therapy (SLT).

F. When to refer to SLT:

1. Speech and voice characteristics are detracting from the message being communicated.

2. Speech and voice are not adequate for daily communication.

3. Speech, voice, and communication problems are interfering with the patient's quality of life.

4. Speech, voice, and communication problems are perceived as troublesome by the patient and family.

■ Dysphagia

A. Normal swallowing involves intricate and rapid coordination of sensory and motor activity in the oral cavity, pharynx, and esophagus.

B. Normal oromotor control for swallowing involves lip closure, facial tone and musculature, rotary lateral jaw motion, and pharyngeal swallow.

C. As a result of MS, the following may occur:

1. A delay in triggering the pharyngeal swallow

2. Difficulty managing thin liquids

3. Problems in the oromotor control phase

4. Reduced tongue coordination

5. Possible esophageal involvement

6. Food aversions due to altered taste sensations

D. Assessment includes a careful history (pneumonia, difficulty with liquids and solids, aspiration, or choking while eating).

E. Optimal management includes referral to a speech–language pathologist familiar with MS and its related problems.

F. Videofluoroscopic examination or modified barium swallow may identify the patient's swallowing pathology. The resulting report should include a description of the patient's physiologic or anatomic swallowing abnormalities, any symptoms associated with the problem, results of any treatment attempted, and recommendations for treatment and dietary intake.

G. Treatment procedures involve the following:

1. Changing the individual's head or body posture

2. Controlling the volume and speed of eating

3. Educating patients and families about voluntary swallowing maneuvers

4. Educating patients and families about fatigue and dysphagia, with advice to rest during long meals and/or to eat more often for a shorter time .

- Sexuality and intimacy

A. Primary sexual dysfunction occurs as a result of MS-related physiologic changes in the central nervous system that directly impact sexual feelings and/or response.

B. Symptoms:

1. Decreased or absent libido

2. Altered genital sensations; decreased frequency, intensity of orgasms

3. Erectile dysfunction

4. Decreased vaginal lubrication, clitoral engorgement

5. Decreased vaginal muscle tone

C. Management

1. Men—pharmacologic management of erectile dysfunction (injections, Levitra, Cialis, and Viagra)

2. Women—medications (lubrication, body mapping assessment)

D. Secondary sexual dysfunction occurs as a result of MS-related physical changes and treatments that indirectly affect sexual feelings and/or response.

E. Etiology

1. Bladder or bowel dysfunction

2. Fatigue

3. Nongenital sensory paresthesias

4. Spasticity

5. Cognitive impairment

6. Tremor, pain

F. Management

1. Treat underlying symptoms

2. Work with symptoms

a. Positioning comfortably

b. Using spasticity to maintain body contact

c. Review and adjust medications

G. Tertiary sexual function is due to psychological, social, and cultural issues that interfere with sexual feelings and/or response. Origins are as follows:

1. Clinical depression

2. Grief

3. Changes in self-image and body image

4. Family and social role changes

5. Anger, guilt, and depression

6. Spousal burden as caregiver

H. Management

1. Counseling of patient and family

2. Grief work

3. Acknowledgment and treatment of intermittent problems

4. Culturally sensitive interventions with appropriate support

I. The nurse's role in working with sexuality and intimacy problems:

1. Evaluate personal attitudes, values, and beliefs

2. Assess personal knowledge

3. Sustain comfort level in patient–partner interaction

J. Some leading questions:

1. Has anything interfered with your ability to maintain closeness?

2. How do you feel about being a man/woman?

3. How has MS changed, if at all, your ability to function sexually?

K. Some sexual assessment tools:

1. The Sexual Health Assessment Framework (Szasz, 1989)

   a. Sexual knowledge

   b. Sexual self-view

   c. Sexual activity

   d. Sexual interest and behavior

   e. Sexual response

2. PLISSIT Model (Annon, 1976)—helps assess for level of intervention for patient

   a. Permission

   b. Limited information

   c. Specific suggestions

   d. Intensive therapy

L. Working with sexuality and intimacy
    1. Open, nonjudgmental atmosphere
    2. Ensure privacy
    3. Encourage open questions
    4. Normalize and validate concerns
    5. Part of the review of systems
    6. Offer resources and reassurance

■ Cognition
    A. The causes of cognitive changes may be divided into primary and secondary effects of the disease.
    B. Primary effects:
        1. The nerve cells themselves.
        2. Lesions are multifocal and vary from person to person in distribution.
        3. This may be explained by cerebral demyelination and axonal damage.
    C. Secondary effects:
        1. Depression
        2. Anxiety
        3. Stress
        4. Fatigue
    D. Frequency, severity, and nature of cognitive changes
        1. Estimates range from 45% to 65% of people with MS having changes.
        2. Only 10% suffer from severe impairment.
        3. No correlation exists between disease course, disease severity, or length of time since diagnosis.
        4. In most cases, cognitive dysfunction is characterized by selective impairment of some functions with relative preservation of others.
        5. Cognitive functions thought to be affected:
            a. Memory (working memory and secondary memory)
            b. Abstract reasoning and problem solving
            c. Attention and concentration (especially sustained or complex attention)
            d. Speed of information processing
            e. Verbal fluency
    E. What is seen clinically?
        1. Inability to think

  2. Inability to remember
  3. Inability to reason logically
F. The nurse's role is to:
  1. Establish a relationship with patients and families
  2. Facilitate communication
  3. Observe and assess
  4. Initiate referrals
  5. Promote coping strategies
  6. Monitor for safety
G. Impact of cognitive impairment
  1. Role strain
    a. Social roles
    b. Work roles
H. Evaluation of cognitive impairment
  1. Informal evaluation
    a. Tool selection
    b. Nursing assessment
  2. Formal neuropsychologic evaluation by neuropsychologists
    a. Patient selection
    b. Patient support
  3. Cognitive rehabilitation (mediocre results)
  4. Potential benefit from disease-modifying agents
  5. Nursing interventions
    a. Recognizing and acknowledging deficits
    b. Accurate report of evaluation results
    c. Patient and family support

■ Depression
A. Disorders of mood and affect
  1. Major depression (subsyndromal depression, suicide is 7.5% greater than general population)
  2. Bipolar affective disorder
  3. Euphoria
  4. Pathologic laughing and crying (mood swings)
B. Major depression
  1. Lifetime in approximately 50% with MS

    2. Point prevalence approximately 14%

    3. Increased compared with other neurologic disorders

C. At risk for depression

    1. Female

    2. Newly diagnosed

    3. Younger age group

D. Possible causes and contributors to depression in MS

    1. Disease activity (especially exacerbations)

    2. Neuropathologic changes in areas of the brain concerned with affective states

    3. Neuroendocrine or psychoneuroimmunologic changes

    4. Reaction to altered life circumstances

    5. Medication side effects

E. Assessment of depression should be done on a regular basis

F. Tools = Center for Epidemiologic Studies Depression Scale, Zung Depression Scale, or Beck Depression Inventory (preferred via consensus)

G. Treatment of depression

    1. Counseling and emotional support, psychotherapy

    2. Pharmacologic management

       a. Tricyclic antidepressants

       b. Mood stabilizing agents such as divalproex sodium (Depakote), lithium carbonate

       c. SSRIs (fluoxetine, sertraline, paroxetine, venlafaxine)

       d. St. John's wort (complementary or alternative medication)

       e. Support and therapeutic groups

■ Nursing care

A. Empowers patients with knowledge and skills development

B. Assists patients to make informed decisions

C. Establishes an interdependent trusting relationship

D. Encourages patients to share expectations, desires, and values

E. Contributes to health-related quality of life (QoL) in MS

    1. Health-related quality of life is a state of complete well-being, and not merely the absence of disease/infirmity.

    2. It is degree of satisfaction with perceived present life circumstances.

    3. It is the perception of the impact of the disease both subjectively and objectively.

4. It is a multidimensional construct emphasizing perceptions.
5. MS has an effect on QoL through its array of symptomatology. Disease disruption ranges from mild to severe and may vary over time according to disease course and available supports.
6. Specific issues related to multiple sclerosis quality of life (MSQoL):
    a. Alterations in social environment
    b. Role reversals in family relationships
    c. Social and emotional isolation
    d. Misinterpretation of symptoms by others
    e. Restricted range of opportunities
    f. Alterations in body image
    g. Impact upon intimate relationships
7. Roles of the nurse in MSQoL
    a. Facilitating adjustment to MS
    b. Establishing a comfortable relationship
    c. Providing education and information
    d. Supporting, empathizing, and "cheerleading"
    e. Communicating, collaborating, and creating
    f. Assisting with adjustment during the postdiagnosis period and throughout lifetime
    g. Empowering patients through self-determination and self-advocacy
    h. Simply being there when needed
8. Strategies to maintain MSQoL
    a. Encompass the patient's ability to:
        i. Adapt
        ii. Communicate
        iii. Socialize
        iv. Be productive
    b. Adapt
        i. Responding to change
        ii. Identifying and evaluating options
        iii. Setting, resetting, and achieving flexible goals
    c. Ability to communicate
        i. Developing and maintaining satisfying relationships
        ii. Determining whether changes are needed in relationships
        iii. Seeking supportive and reciprocal relationships

    d. Ability to be productive

        i. Contributing to homework, school, or volunteer activities

        ii. Feeling that one's opinions matter to others

        iii. Participating in meaningful activities

  9. Significance when patients are cognitively impaired:

    a. Importance of selecting the right style of education

    b. Memory aids to help at home

    c. Frequent follow-up

    d. Reinforcement of actual expectations

    e. Ongoing education of patient/family working with the MS team

RESOURCES

Annon, J. S. (1976). The PLISSIT model: A proposed conceptual scheme for the behavioral treatment of sexual problems. *Journal of Sex Education and Therapy, 2*, 1–15.

Bennett, S. E., Bethoux, F., Brown, T. R., Finlayson, M., Foley, F. W., Heyman, R., & Weinstock-Guttman, B. (2014). Complex symptoms and mobility in multiple sclerosis. *International Journal of MS Care, 16*(Suppl. 1), 1–40.

Ben-Zacharia, A. B. (2011). Therapeutics for multiple sclerosis symptoms. *Mount Sinai Journal of Medicine, 78(2)*, 176–191.

Braley, T. J., & Chervin, R. D. (2010). Fatigue in multiple sclerosis: Mechanisms, evaluation, and treatment. *Sleep, 33*(8), 1061–1067.

Burks, J. S., & Johnson, K. P. (2011). *Multiple sclerosis: Diagnosis, medical management, and rehabilitation.* New York, NY: Demos Medical.

CenterWatch. *Drug information: Ampyra (dalfampridine).* Boston, MA: Author. Retrieved from www.centerwatch.com/drug-information/fda-approvals/drug-details.aspx?DrugID=1080

Cohen, B. A. (2008). Identification, causation, alleviation, and prevention of complications (ICAP): An approach to symptom and disability management in multiple sclerosis. *Neurology, 71*(24, Suppl. 3), S14–S20.

Costello, K., & Halper, J. (2010a). *Multiple sclerosis: Key issues in nursing management: Adherence, cognition, quality of life.* New York, NY: Bioscience.

Costello, K., & Halper, J. (2010b). *Advanced practice nursing in multiple sclerosis: Advanced skills, advancing responsibilities.* Washington, DC: EME.

Di Fabio, R. P., Soderberg, J., Choi, T., Hansen, C. R., & Schapiro, R. T. (1998). Extended outpatient rehabilitation: Its influence on symptom frequency, fatigue, and functional status for persons with progressive multiple sclerosis. *Archives of Physical Medicine and Rehabilitation, 79*, 141–146.

Goodman, A. D., Brown, T. R., Cohen, J. A., Krupp, L.B., Schapiro, R., & Schwid, S. R. (2008). Dose comparison trial of sustained-release fampridine in multiple sclerosis. *Neurology, 71*(15), 1134–1141.

Halper, J. (Ed.). (2007). Advanced symptom management. In J. Halper (Ed.), *Advanced concepts in multiple sclerosis nursing care* (pp. 135–240). New York, NY: Demos Medical.

Halper, J., & Holland, N. J. (Eds.). (2011). *Comprehensive nursing care in multiple sclerosis* (3rd ed.). New York, NY: Springer Publishing Company.

Harris, C., & Halper, J. (2008). *Best practices in nursing care: Disease management, pharmacological treatment, nursing research.* New York, NY: Bioscience.

Hasselkorn, J. K., Balsdon, R. C., Fry, W. D., Herndon, R. M., Johnson, B., Little, J. W., . . . Seidle, M. E. (2005). Overview of spasticity management in multiple sclerosis: Evidence-based management strategies for spasticity treatment in multiple sclerosis. *Journal of Spinal Cord Medicine, 28,* 173–197.

Holland, N. J., & Halper, J. (Eds.). (2005). *Multiple sclerosis: A self-care guide to wellness.* New York, NY: Demos Medical Publishing.

Kachuk, N. J. (2009). Sustained release oral fampridine in the treatment of multiple sclerosis. *Expert Opinion Pharmacotherapeutics, 10*(12), 2025–2035.

Kennedy, P. M. (2011). Incorporating complementary and alternative medicine into symptom management. In J. Halper & N. J. Holland (Eds.), *Comprehensive nursing care in multiple sclerosis* (pp. 123–130). New York, NY: Springer Publishing.

Kinnman, J., Andersson, U., Kinnman, Y., & Wetterqvist, L. (1997). Temporary improvement of motor function in patients with multiple sclerosis after treatment with a cooling suit. *Journal of Neurologic Rehabilitation, 11,* 109–114.

Koch, M., Uyttenboogaart, M., van Harten, A., Heerings, M., & De Keyser, J. (2008). Fatigue, depression, and progression in multiple sclerosis. *Multiple Sclerosis, 14*(6), 815–822.

Messinis, L., Kosmidis, M. H., Lyros, E., & Papathanasopoulos, P. (2010). Assessment and rehabilitation of cognitive impairment in multiple sclerosis. *International Review of Psychiatry, 22,* 22–34.

Namey, M. A. (2011). Managing elimination dysfunction. In J. Halper & N. J. Holland (Eds.), *Comprehensive nursing care in multiple sclerosis* (pp. 31–86). New York, NY: Springer Publishing Company.

Norton, C., & Chelvanayagam, S. (2010). Bowel problems and coping strategies in people with multiple sclerosis. *British Journal of Nursing, 19,* 220–226.

Rae-Grant, A. D., Fox, R. J., Bethoux, F. (Eds). (2013). *Multiple sclerosis and related disorders: Clinical guide to diagnosis, medical management, and rehabilitation.* New York, NY: Demos Medical.

Samkoff, L. M., & Goodman, A. D. (2011). Symptomatic management in multiple sclerosis. *Neurologic Clinics, 29*(2), 449–463.

Schapiro, R. T. (2014). *Managing the symptoms of multiple sclerosis* (6th ed.) New York, NY: Demos Medical.

Schapiro, R. T., & Schneider, D. M. (2011). Managing and minimizing symptoms. In J. Halper & N. J. Holland (Eds.), *Comprehensive nursing care in multiple sclerosis* (pp. 61–86). New York, NY: Springer Publishing Company.

Souza, A., Kelleher, A., Cooper, R., Cooper, R. A., Iezzoni, L. I., & Collins, D. M. (2010). Multiple sclerosis and mobility-related assistive technology: Systematic review of literature. *Journal of Rehabilitation Research and Development, 47,* 213–223.

Szasz, G. (1989). Sexuality in persons with severe physical disability: A guide to the physician. *Canadian Family Physician, 35,* 345–351.

12

The Patient and the Multiple Sclerosis Care Team

OBJECTIVES

Upon completion of this chapter, the learner will be able to:

■ Describe the key participants in the multiple sclerosis (MS) team
■ Discuss the role(s) of rehabilitation specialists in MS
■ Specify the role of the nursing professional in MS as part of the rehabilitation team
■ Identify basic concepts of shared decision making and its relevance to MS

In a disease such as multiple sclerosis (MS), baseline assessments are critical to facilitate monitoring for change and treatment outcomes. These authors would like to emphasize how important it is to obtain a baseline rehabilitation assessment once the patient is diagnosed with MS. This will facilitate planning and monitoring of outcomes throughout the spectrum of the disease.

■ When is rehabilitation provided in MS?
  A. Acutely—during and following exacerbations
  B. Episodically—when functional status changes occur

C. Maintenance—ongoing strategies to sustain function and prevent injury and trauma

- Rehabilitation sites
  A. Inpatient facilities (acute and subacute)
  B. Outpatient care
  C. Home care
  D. Community support programs
  E. Exercise and fitness programs
  F. Wellness programs
  G. Long-term care facilities
  H. Community centers

- The MS rehabilitation team
  A. Patient and family
  B. Physical therapists—ambulation, strengthening, gait, balance, transfers, safety
  C. Occupational therapists—assistive devices, upper extremity function, safety, activities of daily living (ADL)
  D. Speech–language pathologists—speech and swallowing disorders
  E. Neurologists—diagnosis, ongoing management and assessment
  F. Physiatrists (physicians who specialize in rehabilitation medicine)
  G. Nursing professionals—assessment, planning, implementation, coordination
  H. Ophthalmologists (neuro-ophthalmologists)—visual problems related to MS
  I. Psychologists—emotional issues related to adjustment to MS
  J. Neuropsychologists—cognitive challenges
  K. Social workers—environmental, social, and emotional adjustment
  L. Vocational specialists—employment issues
  M. Clergy—spiritual needs
  N. Case managers—reimbursement issues for necessary care
  O. Community advocacy organizations (see www.multiplesclerosis coalition.org)

- Adapting to change
  A. Functional status
  B. Assistive devices
  C. Educational needs

D. Environmental modifications

E. Vocational rehabilitation

F. Economic concerns

G. Long-term planning

- Supporting the family throughout the spectrum of MS
  A. Counseling
  B. Education
  C. Emotional support
  D. Ongoing communication
  E. Advocacy
  F. Setting realistic and achievable goals
  G. Supporting needed changes

- Principles of neurorehabilitation in MS
  A. Should be dynamic, flexible, and creative.
  B. Issues such as patient and family financial status, insurance coverage, history of adherence, cognitive impairment and its effect on learning, and quality of life should be considered when planning and implementing new strategies and using new techniques.
  C. Neurorehabilitation in MS requires a team approach, with collaboration among the team, the patient, and the family.
  D. As stated earlier, considerations in neurorehabilitation include the following:
     1. Extent of insurance coverage
     2. Family and social support
     3. Patient's residential, social, cultural, and economic environment
     4. Ability to participate in and carry out treatment plan

- Supporting transitions in MS (new diagnosis, relapses, progression)
  A. Acknowledge the problems.
  B. Refer the patient to appropriate resources.
  C. Assist with access to adequate services.
  D. Coach, partner, and reassure.
  E. Reevaluate on a regular basis.

- Empowerment
  A. Empower using:
     1. Modeling

2. Assessment and teaching tools

3. Environmental and lifestyle modifications

4. Patient and family education

5. Support

6. Encouragement of shared decision making and self-efficacy (see references and resources listed at the end of this chapter).

   a. Shared decision making—important to consider when dealing with issues related to a long-term, chronic disease.

   b. Shared decision making is the collaboration between patients and caregivers to come to an agreement about a health care decision. It is especially useful when there is no clear "best" treatment option.

   c. Enables patients and families to take control of problems through active participation.

   d. Equal input from both patient and professional.

   e. Information sharing and communication essential.

RESOURCES

Bennett, S. E., Bethoux, F., Brown, T. R., Finlayson, M., Foley, F. W., Heyman, R., & Weinstock-Guttman, B. (2014). Complex symptoms and mobility in multiple sclerosis. *International Journal of MS Care, 16*(Suppl. 1), 1–40.

Bennett, S. E., Bobryk, P., Bednarik, P., & Smith, C. (2015). *A practical guide to rehabilitation in multiple sclerosis.* Old Lyme, CT: The France Foundation.

Bethoux, F., & McKee, K. (2013). Multiple sclerosis and ambulation. In A. D. Rae Grant, R. J. Fox, & F. Bethoux (Eds.), *Multiple sclerosis and related disorders* (pp. 226–234). New York, NY: Demos Medical Publishing.

Burks, J. S., Bigley, G. K., & Hill, H. H. (2009). Rehabilitation challenges in multiple sclerosis. *Annals of Indian Academy of Neurology, 12,* 296–306.

Carpiac-Claver, M., Guzman, J. S., & Castle, S. C. (2007). The comprehensive care clinic. *Health and Social Work, 32*(3), 220–223.

Dalgas, U., Stenager, E., Jakobsen, J., Petersen, T., Hansen, H. J., Knudsen, C., . . . Ingemann-Hansen, T. (2010). Fatigue, mood and quality of life improve in MS patients after progressive resistance training. *Multiple Sclerosis, 16,* 480–490.

Dartmouth-Hitchcock. (n.d.). *Shared decision making* (Courtesy of the High Value Healthcare Collaborative—Dartmouth Institute for Health Policy & Clinical Practice). Lebanon, NH: Author. Retrieved from www.dartmouth-hitchcock .org/medical-information/decision_making_help.html

Fraser, R., Johnson, E., Ehde, D., & Bishop, M. (n.d.). *Patient self-management in multiple sclerosis.* Retrieved from University of Washington Multiple Sclerosis Rehabilitation Research and Training Center website: http://msrrtc .washington.edu/resources/CMSC_WhitePaper.pdf

Halper, J. (2008). Comprehensive care in multiple sclerosis—A patient-centered approach. *European Neurology, 3,* 72–74.

Hobart, J. C., Riazi, A., Lamping, D. L., Fitzpatrick, R., & Thompson, A. J. (2005). How responsive is the Multiple Sclerosis Impact Scale (MSIS-29)? A comparison with some other self report scales. *Journal of Neurology, Neurosurgery and Psychiatry, 76*(11), 1539–1543.

Kalb, R. (2012). *Multiple sclerosis: A focus on rehabilitation* (5th ed.). New York, NY: National Multiple Sclerosis Society. Retrieved from www.nationalmssociety. org/for-professionals/download.aspx?id=22556

Kennedy, P. (2011). Collaborating with the rehabilitation team. In J. Halper & N. J. Holland (Eds.), *Comprehensive nursing care in multiple sclerosis* (3rd ed., pp. 215–236). New York, NY: Springer Publishing Company.

Lisak, R. P., & Korngold, S. (2010). Insights for practice: Where mechanism of action meets patient management. *Neurology, 74*(Suppl. 1), S70–S73.

McCullagh, R., Fitzgerald, A. P., Murphy, R. P., & Mater, G. C. (2008). Long-term benefits of exercising on quality of life and fatigue in multiple sclerosis patients with mild disability: A pilot study. *Clinical Rehabilitation, 22*(3), 206–214.

Motl, R. W., McAuley, E., & Snook, M. (2005). Physical activity and multiple sclerosis: A meta-analysis. *Multiple Sclerosis, 11,* 459–463.

Petajan, E. T., Gappmaier, E., White, A. T., Spencer, M. K., Mino, L., & Hicks, R. W. (1996). Impact of aerobic training on fitness and quality of life in multiple sclerosis. *Annals of Neurology, 39,* 432–441.

Provance, P. G. (2008). *Physical therapy in multiple sclerosis rehabilitation* (clinical bulletin). New York, NY: National Multiple Sclerosis Society. Retrieved from www.nationalmssociety.org/download.aspx?id=163

Provance, P. G. (2010). *Rehabilitation philosophy in MS care.* Presented at the Consortium of Multiple Sclerosis Centers 2010 Annual Meeting. Retrieved from http://iomsrt.mscare.org/clinical-page/slide-presentations

Rabow, M. W., Dibble, S. L., Pantilat, S. Z., & McPhee, S. J. (2004). The comprehensive care team. *Archives of Internal Medicine, 164,* 83–91.

Rietberg, M. B., Brooks, D., Uitdehaag, B. M. J., & Kwakkel, G. (2005). Exercise therapy for multiple sclerosis. *Cochrane Database Systematic Reviews, 1,* CD003980. Retrieved from www.cochrane.org

Schapiro, R. T. (2014). *Symptom management in multiple sclerosis* (6th ed.). New York, NY: Demos Medical.

13

Bladder Dysfunction in Multiple Sclerosis

OBJECTIVES

Upon completion of this chapter, the learner will be able to:

- Describe the anatomy and physiology of the urinary tract
- Identify the neurologic innervation of the urinary tract
- Cite the diagnostic procedures used in the assessment of urinary dysfunction in multiple sclerosis (MS)
- Discuss preventative measures and optimal management of urinary dysfunction in MS
- Describe the nursing role using comprehensive strategies

Approximately 80% of patients with multiple sclerosis (MS) experience significant bladder dysfunction at some point during the course of their disease. Bladder dysfunction causes alterations in personal, social, and vocational activities, along with sleep disruption, embarrassment, dependency, and isolation. Nursing plays a major role in the assessment and treatment of bladder dysfunction. The nurse can help the individual with MS achieve a predictable and effective elimination plan and minimize complications.

■ Treatment goals

A. Maintain renal function

B. Maintain continence

C. Establish normal voiding patterns

D. Reduce symptoms and improve quality of life

E. Motivate patient to adhere to treatment

F. Educate patient to promote a wellness lifestyle

■ Normal urinary function

A. The kidneys of an adult female produce 100 to 125 mL/hr.

B. Males produce about 150 mL/hr.

C. The actual rate depends on fluid intake, position, and kidney function.

D. Kidneys produce urine more efficiently in the supine position.

E. Ureters are thin-walled muscular tubes that move urine from the kidneys to the bladder.

F. Closure of the ureters during bladder contraction is accomplished by contraction of the trigone area during voiding.

G. The main function of the urinary bladder is to store and expel urine.

H. The bladder is a hollow muscular organ that is supported by loose connective tissue. The trigone and lower portion of the base of the bladder rest upon the anterior vaginal wall in women. The wall of the bladder consists of an inner mucous membrane with a cell lining and underlying lamina propria; a layer of smoother muscle, the detrusor; and an outer layer of connective tissue.

I. The urethra has an internal and external sphincter mechanism. The interior sphincter has three components (urethral mucosa, periurethral connective tissue, and periurethral vascular plexus). Each is responsible for one-third of the urethral closure pressure. The internal sphincter is composed of small muscle bundles and is not under voluntary control. The external sphincter is under voluntary control.

J. The bladder is innervated by sympathetic fibers from the hypogastric nerve at T10 through L2 and parasympathetic fibers from the pelvic nerve at S2 through S4.

K. As the bladder fills with urine, its fundus rises into the lower abdominal cavity.

L. To initiate voiding, the urethra relaxes first, then the bladder contracts and expels the urine through the relaxed sphincter. These functions occur automatically.

M. Average bladder capacity for an adult is 300 to 500 mL. The initial urge to void occurs when approximately 200 mL has accumulated. Contractions of the bladder are inhibited by the nervous system until 300 mL has been collected. An individual can sense bladder fullness and can initiate or postpone emptying as convenient.

N. Normally, a person voids four to six times during a 24-hour period, depending on fluid intake, type, and amount.

■ Bladder dysfunction problems occurring in MS
Bladder symptoms may be explained in terms of failure to store urine (storage symptoms) and/or failure to empty (voiding and postmicturition symptoms).

A. Bladder dysfunction in MS is primarily associated with demyelination in the spinal cord, the pontine cerebellar micturition control areas, or other central nervous system points in between.

B. Interruption of the spinal cord pathways may result in excessive detrusor contractions, involuntary sphincter relaxation or contraction, or detrusor areflexia with urinary retention.

C. Bladder dysfunction, or neurogenic bladder, may produce the following:

1. Urinary urgency—a strong need to urinate that cannot be controlled or postponed.

2. Urinary frequency—the need to urinate more often than every 2 to 3 hours.

3. Urinary hesitancy—difficulty initiating the flow of urine.

4. Nocturia—waking up more than once during the night to urinate.

5. Incontinence—losing control of urine.

6. Incomplete emptying—feeling that some urine is left in the bladder after urinating.

7. Urinary tract infections (UTIs)—resulting in classic symptoms of burning or pain upon urination. This may result in a temporary worsening of MS symptoms or may be the first sign that a person is experiencing a change in usual bladder function.

D. The presence of one or more of these symptoms is suggestive of a neurogenic bladder.

E. The three common types of bladder dysfunction are the result of the following:

1. Hypercontractility of the detrusor muscle

2. Inability of the sphincter to relax and open, or detrusor areflexia

3. Incoordination of the detrusor and sphincter activity: detrusor-sphincter dyssynergia (DSD)

    F. In summary, bladder dysfunction in MS can result in failure to store urine, failure to empty urine, or combined dysfunction.

    G. Similar symptoms may be present in all three types of bladder dysfunction.

■ Assessment of bladder dysfunction

    A. Evaluation of patient's chief concern

    B. History of voiding pattern, daytime and nighttime

    C. History of incontinent episodes

    D. Urinary patterns and symptoms—urgency, frequency, incontinence, hesitancy, hematuria, use of protective pads, dysuria, UTIs

    E. Medical history—abdominal surgery, number of full-term pregnancies, gynecologic problems

    F. Current medications

    G. Evaluation of postvoid residual via straight catheterization or bladder ultrasound

        1. In straight catheterization, patient drinks two 8-oz glasses of water prior to assessment.

        a. Patient voids, and output is measured.

        b. Patient is catheterized for postvoid residual urine.

        c. Greater than 100 mL, the patient requires instruction in self-catheterization.

        d. Frequency of self-catheterization depends on the amount of urine remaining in the bladder after voiding.

        e. If there is 100 mL in the bladder, can be done once daily.

        f. If more than 200 mL, twice daily.

        g. If residual is less than 60 mL, patient is prescribed medications to control or reduce bladder spasms and promote more efficient bladder storage of urine.

    H. Bladder ultrasound

        1. Full bladder is scanned for total volume of urine in bladder.

        2. Patient voids.

        3. Bladder is rescanned to determine postvoid residual.

    I. Intervention is the same as described in G

    J. With intermittent self-catheterization (ISC) in the case of a failure-to-empty bladder, the addition of anticholinergic or antimuscarinic medication may be considered to reduce patient's symptoms despite fully emptying the bladder

■ Additional studies

A. Kidney and bladder ultrasound can yield information about structural abnormalities causing symptoms.

B. Intravenous pyelogram can outline the ureters and is also a test of kidney function.

C. Urodynamic studies clarify the function of the muscles of the lower urinary tract. Complete urodynamic testing includes uroflowmetry, the quantitative and qualitative analysis of urinary stream. It is the measurement of the rate of urination and force of the bladder's expulsive ability.

D. Pressure flow parameters in the study include bladder pressure, rectal pressure, differential pressure, urethral pressure, flow rate, volume, and electromyogram sphincter activity.

E. Both needle and surface electromyogram and CMG (filling cys-tometrogram) are helpful in diagnosing DSD.

■ Bladder management interventions

A. Bladder training consists of education, scheduled voiding, and positive reinforcement. This requires that the participant resist or inhibit the sensation of urgency to postpone voiding and urinate according to a timetable rather than according to the urge to void.

B. Bladder training may also involve tactics to allow the bladder to hold a greater volume.

1. Drinking an adequate amount of fluid at one sitting will generally result in an urge to void within the retraining time frame.

2. Avoiding fluids with caffeine, artificial sweeteners, and alcohol will reduce bladder irritability.

3. Protective pads may absorb involuntary urine outflow.

4. Male external catheters may help do the same.

5. Medications that are beneficial for failure to store and DSD include the following:

   a. Anticholinergics (oxybutynin)

   b. Antimuscarinics (tolterodine tartrate, hyoscyamine sulfate)

   c. Tricyclic antidepressants (imipramine)

   d. Antidiuretic hormone analog (desmopressin acetate), particularly for nocturia

C. Crede method is contraindicated because of the potential to create increased pressure and thereby damage the upper tract.

D. Kegel exercises and pelvic floor muscle therapy may be recommended.

E. Intermittent self-catheterization.

1. Allows an individual to empty the bladder at regular intervals, thereby reducing the risk of UTI, structural damage, and other distressing bladder symptoms.

2. This technique has been widely supported in the literature. It uses a clean technique. Teaching guides are available.

F. An indwelling catheter may be needed for either short- or long-term use and allows for continual drainage by gravity.

1. Its use is suggested for those individuals who cannot be managed with ISC and/or medications or who have a chronic decubitus ulcer and cannot perform ISC.

2. Long-term use of indwelling catheters is a significant source of bacteruria and UTI. Management varies, but the usual practice is to change the catheter after a minimum of 30 days or pro re nata (PRN). If the patient has a symptomatic UTI, the entire system must be changed and a urine culture obtained.

3. A person with MS may still experience urinary incontinence with an indwelling catheter. In this instance, the indication is not to increase the size of the catheter or balloon, but rather to use anticholinergic/antimuscarinic medications to decrease urinary tract spasticity.

4. When bladder symptoms do not improve, referral to a urologist is recommended.

5. Patients may be candidates for other treatment strategies, including Botox (onabotulinum-toxin A) injections or other complex procedures designed to facilitate urinary continence. Additional information is available at www.uspharmacist.com/continuing_education/ceviewtest/lessonid/110329.

■ Surgical interventions

A. Suprapubic catheters are an alternative to long-term urethral catheters. These may be helpful in male patients and in women who have developed severe urethral irritation secondary to an indwelling Foley catheter.

B. Sphincterectomy may be recommended for very disabled male patients who experience intractable hesitancy and retention. Anticholinergic medications and an external condom catheter can be combined to manage bladder activity.

C. Some female patients with small-capacity bladder may benefit from a laparoscopic procedure that includes bladder augmentation with a continent diversion. Patients can then catheterize a stoma at the navel or abdomen.

D. Diversion procedures include cystostomy or transurethral resection, which provides a clear passageway for the urine to flow freely. This procedure is used only rarely.

RESOURCES

Abrams, P., Cardozo, L., Fall, M., Griffiths, D., Rosier, P., Ulmsten, U., . . . Wein, A. (2002). The standardisation of terminology of lower urinary tract function: report from the Standardisation Sub-committee of the International Continence Society. *Neurourology and Urodynamics, 21*(2), 167–178.

Adigun, M., Adesoye, A., Ayoola, A., Lteif, L., & Amaechi, O. (2014, August). *Review of nonneurogenic overactive bladder.* Retrieved from www.uspharmacist .com/continuing_education/ceviewtest/lessonid/110329

Araki, I., Matsui, M., Ozawa, K., Takeda, M., & Kuno, S. (2003). Relationship of bladder dysfunction to lesion site in multiple sclerosis. *Journal of Urology, 169*(4), 1384–1387. doi:10.1097/01.ju.0000049644.27713.c8

Ciancio, S. J., Mutchnik, S. E., Rivera, V. M., & Boone, T. B. (2001). Urodynamic pattern changes in multiple sclerosis. *Urology, 57*(2), 239–245.

Crayton, H., Heyman, R. A., & Rossman, H. S. (2004). A multimodal approach to managing the symptoms of multiple sclerosis. *Neurology, 63*(11, Suppl. 5), S12–S18.

Cutter, G. R., Zimmerman, J., Salter, A. R., Knappertz, V., Suarez, G., Waterbor, J., . . . Marrie, R. A. (2015). Causes of death among persons with multiple sclerosis. *Multiple Sclerosis and Related Disorders, 4*(5), 484–490. doi:10.1016/ j. msard.2015.07.008

De Sèze, M., Ruffion, A., Denys, P., Joseph, P.-A., & Perrouin-Verbe, B.; GENULF. (2007). The neurogenic bladder in multiple sclerosis: Review of the literature and proposal of management guidelines. *Multiple Sclerosis (Houndmills, Basingstoke, England), 13*(7), 915–928. doi:10.1177/1352458506075651

Elimination dysfunction in multiple sclerosis. (2012). *International Journal of MS Care, 14*(Suppl. 1), 1–26. doi:10.7224/1537-2073-14.S1.1

Giannantoni, A., Scivoletto, G., Di Stasi, S. M., Grasso, M. G., Finazzi Agrò, E., Collura, G., & Vespasiani, G. (1999). Lower urinary tract dysfunction and disability status in patients with multiple sclerosis. *Archives of Physical Medicine and Rehabilitation, 80*(4), 437–441.

Mahajan, S. T., Patel, P. B., & Marrie, R. A. (2010). Undertreatment of overactive bladder symptoms in patients with multiple sclerosis: An ancillary analysis of the NARCOMS Patient Registry. *Journal of Urology, 183*(4), 1432–1437. doi:10.1016/j.juro.2009.12.029

National Multiple Sclerosis Society. (2015). *Bladder problems.* New York, NY: Author. Retrieved from National MS Society website: www.nationalmssociety .org/Symptoms-Diagnosis/MS-Symptoms/Bladder-Dysfunction

Orasanu, B., & Mahajan, S. T. (2013). Bladder and bowel dysfunction in multiple sclerosis. In A. D. Rae-Grant, R. J. Fox, & F. Bethoux (Eds.), *Multiple sclerosis and related disorders* (pp. 200–210). New York, NY: Demos Medical.

14

Bowel Elimination and Continence

OBJECTIVES

Upon completion of this chapter, the learner will be able to:

- *Identify the common pathophysiology of upper motor neuron bowel, lower motor neuron bowel, uninhibited neurogenic bowel, and motor paralytic bowel as seen in multiple sclerosis (MS)*
- *Identify desired outcomes of a bowel program in MS*
- *Identify common nursing interventions in managing a neurogenic bowel*
- *Create a comprehensive care plan for gastrointestinal complication*

Altered bowel function may occur whenever the central nervous system has been impaired. When disease or disability results in altered bowel control, incontinence may become as devastating a problem as the disease itself. Control of incontinence and prevention of constipation and diarrhea are possible through an effective bowel program, which requires knowledge of normal and altered bowel physiology and an in-depth assessment of bowel function.

- Normal bowel anatomy and physiology
    A. The lower bowel acts under voluntary control to store and eliminate feces.

B. Inability to store fecal matter causes problems with involuntary bowel or incontinence.

C. Inability to eliminate causes constipation.

D. The bowel consists of three separate parts: the ileum, the cecum, and the colon.

E. The ileum is approximately the last third of the small intestine.

   1. It is approximately 12 ft long and extends from the jejunum to the ileocecal opening.

   2. Almost all absorption and digestion are accomplished in the small intestine.

   3. The small intestine absorbs water and sodium and secretes mucus, potassium, and bicarbonate for stool formation.

F. The cecum is 6 cm in length and lies below the terminal ileum, forming the first part of the large intestine.

G. The colon is the division of the large intestine that extends from the cecum to the rectum.

   1. In the colon, fluids and electrolytes are reabsorbed and feces are stored so that defecation can occur at an acceptable time.

   2. Defecation is affected by peristalsis, anorectal sensory awareness, anal sphincter function, and abdominal muscle function and strength.

H. The rectum is the 12-cm segment of the large bowel between the sigmoid colon and the anal canal. As a rule, it does not contain feces except during defecation.

I. The anal canal comprises the last 3 cm of the digestive tubes. Striated muscle in the anal canal and pelvic floor provides support to the rectal wall and anus, thus maintaining continence.

■ Neurogenic bowel

A. Constipation

   1. Neurogenic bowel results from the interruption of neural pathways that supply the rectum, external sphincter, and accessory muscles involved in defecation.

   2. Nerve impulses that are disrupted may impede cerebral recognition of anal contents and the need to empty stool at a desired or planned time.

   3. Slowed transit may result in constipation.

   4. Weakened abdominal muscles may make bearing down very difficult.

5. Decreased activity related to altered mobility, fatigue, or a sedentary lifestyle may contribute to slow bowel function.

6. Constipation has been defined as less than or equal to two bowel movements per week, or the need for stimulation or the use of laxatives, enemas, or suppositories more than once a week.

7. Constipation has also been characterized by hard, dry stool, causing straining or painful defecation and resulting in a delay of passage of food residue.

8. Medications contributing to constipation may include the following:

   a. Analgesics
   b. Anticholinergics
   c. Anticonvulsants
   d. Antidepressants
   e. Diuretics
   f. Psychotherapeutics
   g. Iron
   h. Opiates
   i. Muscle relaxants

9. Other factors that contribute to neurogenic bowel conditions:

   a. Inadequate or lack of exercise
   b. Limited fluid intake
   c. Reduced intake of dietary fiber
   d. Effects of medications

B. Diarrhea or involuntary bowel

1. Diarrhea may result from gastrointestinal influenza, dietary irritants, and gastrointestinal disorders.

2. Diarrhea (loose, liquid stools) and frequent discharge of fluid fecal matter may be secondary to:

   a. Fecal impaction
   b. Diet or irritating foods
   c. Inflammation or irritation of the bowel
   d. Stress, anxiety
   e. Medications
   f. Overuse of laxatives or stool softeners
   g. Dietary intolerance of milk products, chocolate

    3. Diarrhea may be accompanied by urgency, cramping, abdominal pain, increased bowel sounds, or increased volume of stools.

    4. In multiple sclerosis (MS), involuntary bowel or fecal incontinence is the result of interruption in the neural pathways and impaired cortical awareness of the urge to defecate.

       a. Characterized by urgency and involuntary stools

       b. Defecation is sudden with or without urgency

       c. Patient may also experience partial or total sensory loss in the perineum and rectum

       d. Assessment and management of bowel function/dysfunction

C. Questions to ask include the use of medications that influence bowel activity, such as diuretics, antacids, nonsteroidal anti-inflammatory agents, anticholinergics, antidepressants, antibiotics, laxatives, and enemas.

    1. Presence or absence of the awareness of the need to defecate

    2. Frequency and quality of stool, including color and consistency

    3. Fluid and dietary history should include fluid intake, daily intake of fiber, and type of food or snacks eaten

    4. Objective assessment of the abdomen should include auscultation, palpation, and percussion

    5. Assessment should include patient's functional ability to ambulate and transfer, the use of assistive devices, the ability to remove clothing, and the accessibility of toilet facilities

D. Interventions to manage bowel dysfunction:

    1. Goals of bowel training program include:

       a. Normalizing stool consistency

       b. Establishing a regular pattern for defecation

       c. Stimulating rectal emptying on a routine basis

       d. Avoiding complications of diarrhea, constipation, or incontinence

       e. Improving the patient's quality of life

E. Constipation should first be treated with nonpharmacologic interventions

    1. Increase fluid intake (1.5–2 quarts daily), fiber (20–30 g/day), and exercise.

    2. Education and support are equally important.

    3. Establish a regular pattern of bowel elimination.

    4. Attempt to defecate 1/2 hour after meals when the gastrocolic reflex is the strongest.

    5. Sit in an upright position with feet on the floor.

6. The program may take 3 to 4 weeks or longer.

7. The use of stool softeners or bulk formers with fluids and fiber may help.

8. Oral stimulants provide a chemical stimulation and a localized mechanical stimulation and lubrication to promote elimination of stool.

9. Glycerin suppositories provide lubrication for passage of stool.

10. Medicated suppositories stimulate strong, involuntary, wavelike movement that facilitates the elimination of stool.

11. Regular use of enemas should be avoided to minimize the risk of dependency.

12. Fecal impaction is a complication of chronic constipation. Manual disimpaction or soap suds enemas are the options for immediate treatment, but long-term management using the bowel training program is the appropriate option.

13. An episode of fecal impaction is an indication for an aggressive bowel program.

F. Fecal incontinence

1. Adequate bulk and fiber are important for maintenance of stool consistency. Patients should be instructed to avoid overly spicy and gas-forming foods.

2. Planned times for bowel evacuation and the use of suppositories to stimulate rectal emptying allow for more bowel control.

3. Establishing a routine eliminates involuntary bowel accidents.

4. Encourage the patient to sit on a toilet or commode for 10 to 15 minutes after consuming a hot beverage.

5. The following strategies may help:

a. Sit comfortably on the toilet and try to "bear down."

b. Rocking back and forth and massaging the abdomen can promote bowel activity.

c. If the bowels do not move within 15 minutes, leave the bathroom and try again later when another "urge" is present.

G. Nutritional and fluid intake guidelines

1. Liquid intake should be about 8 to 12 cups or 2,000 mL/d.

2. Be aware that increased liquid intake can be problematic in patients with urinary problems.

3. Avoid or minimize dietary irritants such as caffeine or alcohol.

4. The addition of fiber in the diet can significantly improve stool consistency and decrease transit time. The Recommended Dietary Allowance (RDA) is at least 15 g daily in gradually increasing doses.

    5. If a high-fiber diet cannot be tolerated, bulking agents can be taken with liquid.

    6. Gas and bloating can be avoided by gradually incorporating a sensible balanced diet eaten at regular times.

  H. Expected outcomes of bowel management

    1. Predictable, regular bowel evacuation.

    2. Decrease in episodes of constipation or involuntary bowel.

    3. Formed stool.

    4. Avoidance of prescription drugs, strong laxatives, or enemas.

    5. Patient and family awareness of the elements of bowel management.

    6. Patient and family awareness of early signs of bowel dysfunction.

  I. Medications that relieve constipation

    1. Stimulant laxatives

    2. Fiber supplements/bulk formers

    3. Stool softeners

    4. Osmotically active and saline laxatives

  J. Medications that relieve diarrhea

    1. Antidiarrheals

    2. Bulking agents

RESOURCES

Beadnall, H. N., Kuppananda, K. E., O'Connell, A., Hardy, T. A., Reddel, S. W., & Barnett, M. H. (2015). Tablet-based screening improves continence management in multiple sclerosis. *Annals of Clinical and Translational Neurology, 2*(60), 679–687.

Coggrave, M., Norton, C., & Cody, J. B. (2014). Management of faecal incontinence and constipation in adults with central neurological diseases. *Cochrane Database Systematic Reviews, 1*, CD002115.

Hawker, K. S., & Frohman, E. M. (2001). Bladder, bowel and sexual dysfunction in multiple sclerosis. *Current Treatment Options in Neurology, 3*(3), 207–214. Retrieved from www.springlink.com/content/j41555712143/

Kim, J.-H. (2011). Management of urinary and bowel dysfunction in multiple sclerosis. In B. G. Giesser (Ed.), *Primer on multiple sclerosis* (pp. 197–209). New York, NY: Oxford University Press.

Krogh, K., & Christensen, P. (2009). Neurogenic colorectal and pelvic floor dysfunction. *Best Practice and Research Clinical Gastroenterology, 23,* 531–543.

Namey, M. (2011). Managing elimination dysfunction. In J. Halper & N. Holland (Eds.), *Comprehensive nursing care in multiple sclerosis* (pp. 87–108). New York, NY: Springer Publishing Company.

Patel, D. P., Elliott, S. P., Stoffel, J. T., Brant, W. O., Hotaling, J. M., & Myers, J. B. (2014). Patient reported outcomes measures in neurogenic bladder and bowel: A systematic review of the current literature. *Neurourology and Urodynamics, 35*(1), 8–14.

Saquil, A., Kane, S., & Farnell, E. (2014). Multiple sclerosis: A primary care perspective. *American Family Physician, 90*(9), 644–652.

15

The Nurse's Role in Advanced Multiple Sclerosis

OBJECTIVES

Upon completion of this chapter, the learner will be able to:

- Describe key issues of concern in worsening and/or advanced multiple sclerosis (MS)
- Discuss nursing implications in progressive disease
- Cite specific strategies in avoiding complications of this advanced condition
  - Address physical and emotional implications of worsening disease
  - Describe the psychosocial impact of increasing disability and dependence

- Primary progressive and advanced multiple sclerosis (MS)

  A. A small percentage (5%) of people with MS become severely disabled with increasing symptoms and decreasing function.

  B. Along with altered physical function, emotional and environmental issues become greater challenges.

  C. Professional and personal caregivers are faced with ongoing tasks to meet the special needs in this population.

D. The nurse is challenged as both a care professional and an educator of the patient, family, and responsible others in the patient's life.

■ Nutrition

A. General nutrition

1. A well-balanced diet is important throughout one's lifetime, whether sick or well.

2. Good nutrition is characterized by a well-developed body with ideal weight, healthy hair and skin, and mental alertness.

3. Recommended dietary allowance by the U.S. Department of Agriculture are guidelines for health professionals and patients.

4. Recommendations include servings in bread and cereal group, vegetable and fruit groups, limiting fat intake, and adequate intake of water and fluids.

5. No conclusive evidence suggests that any nutritional therapy affects the course of MS.

6. The nurse is in an excellent position to educate patients and families about nutrition.

7. Dietary supplements and a variety of vitamins, antioxidants, and minerals have made therapeutic claims for benefit, but there is no evidence to support these claims at present.

B. Factors that can affect nutrition

1. Tremor, weakness, paralysis, and dysphagia can interfere with adequate food intake.

2. Fatigue and depression may alter nutritional status.

3. Patient's financial situation may limit access to adequate nutrition.

4. Altered mobility may diminish patient's ability to obtain food staples required for meal preparation and adequate intake.

C. Managing nutritional problems

1. Patient's weight should be monitored.

2. A swallowing evaluation should be recommended when indicated.

3. A registered dietitian can determine caloric needs based on activity level.

4. A person with skin breakdown will need increased calories and protein to promote healing.

5. Feeding techniques and education may be required in a person with dysphagia.

6. Referrals to home health programs to relieve the caregiver may be necessary.

7. Meals on Wheels or food stamps may be helpful.

8. Those with decreased energy may precook or microwave meals.

9. Small, frequent feedings may be recommended.

10. Adaptive equipment such as weighted utensils, elongated straws, and modified dishes may be helpful.

11. Nutritional supplements may ensure adequate intake in patients with fatigue.

12. Fluid intake in advanced MS:

   a. Minimum of eight glasses needed daily (1,500–2,000 mL/24 hours)

   b. Urinary tract infections (UTIs) can be reduced with acidification and hydration

   c. Fluids can be obtained through gelatin and other desserts

   d. Supplemental tube feedings may be necessary

■ Urinary tract infections

A. UTIs pose a serious threat in advanced MS.

B. Urinary drainage may be accomplished through spontaneous voiding, intermittent catheterization, or indwelling catheter.

C. Although intermittent catheterization is the preferred artificial way of emptying the bladder, indwelling catheters are a reality in advanced disease. Chronic, indwelling catheters should be latex-free, made of materials such as silicone or hydrogel.

D. Attention must be given to keeping tubing and drainage bags as clean as possible.

E. Catheters should be changed as needed (i.e., infection or obstruction), regularly.

F. Patients must be monitored for signs and symptoms of UTI (fever, urine analysis, culture and sensitivity test, increased spasticity, etc.).

G. Treatment of UTIs (symptomatic versus colonized) should be initiated promptly.

■ Toileting and personal hygiene

A. Bowel programs become a greater challenge because transferring and environmental barriers cause the need for increased physical care.

B. Families as well as formal caregivers may need more assistance.

C. Costs of personal care increase in view of the need for environmental adaptations and home modifications.

  D. Social services and community support may be required.

  E. Rehabilitation services may be targeted to maintaining safety rather than restorative.

■ Spasticity

  A. Management is a challenge because of intercurrent symptoms such as fatigue and weakness.

  B. Medications consist of baclofen, tizanidine, dantrolene, diazepam, and gabapentin.

  C. Stretching, positioning, and range of motion (ROM) are important to maintain muscle length and tone.

  D. Blocks and surgical techniques may be beneficial.

  E. The advent of intrathecal delivery of baclofen is a breakthrough in the management of intractable spasticity.

  F. Pump maintenance and dose titration are relatively simple.

■ Skin care

  A. Prevention of skin breakdown is essential.

  B. Braden and Norton Scales have been validated in MS.

  C. Braces or splints may cause friction or pressure.

  D. Maintenance of desired weight is important.

  E. Nursing activities include the following:

    1. Identification of predisposing factors

    2. Patient and family education

    3. Use of appropriate assistive devices for transfers

    4. Regular skin inspection

    5. Maintenance of bowel and bladder continence

    6. Adequate personal hygiene

    7. Adequate nutrition and fluid intake

■ Personal care

  A. Formal and informal caregivers may be required.

  B. Respite care is important to prevent burnout.

  C. Alternative long-term solutions may have to be explored.

  D. Day treatment programs may relieve caregiver burden.

■ Family needs

  A. Advanced directives should be discussed.

  B. Life planning should be encouraged.

C. Counseling and education are essential to support family needs.

D. Community agencies are important assets at this time.

E. Opportunities to communicate fears and concerns are important.

F. Discussions about palliative care may enter the dialogue, including discussions about hospice care and community resources.

RESOURCES

Baranzini, S., Bar-Or, A., Cohen, J., Cross, A., Foley, F., Goodman, A., . . . Wingerchuk, D. (2010). Progressive multiple sclerosis: A comprehensive update: Report from a CMSC Consensus Meeting. *International Journal of MS Care, 12*(Suppl. 2), 1–51.

Burks, J., & Johnson, K. (Eds.). (2000). *Multiple sclerosis: Diagnosis, medical management, and rehabilitation.* New York, NY: Demos Medical.

Coyle, P. K., & Halper, J. (2001). *Meeting the challenges of progressive multiple sclerosis.* New York, NY: Demos Medical.

Coyle, P. K., & Halper, J. (2007). *Living with progressive multiple sclerosis.* New York, NY: Demos Medical.

Halper, J. (Ed.). (2007). *Advanced concepts in multiple sclerosis nursing.* New York, NY: Demos Medical.

Harris, C. (2002). Prevention of complications in the severely disabled. In J. Halper & N. Holland (Eds.), *Comprehensive nursing care in multiple sclerosis* (pp. 93–122). New York, NY: Demos Medical.

Lehman, L., & Picone M. A. (2002). Pulmonary complications. In J. Halper (Ed.), *Advanced concepts in multiple sclerosis nursing care* (pp. 137–148), New York, NY: Demos Medical.

Miller, D. H., & Leary, S. M. (2007). Primary-progressive multiple sclerosis. *Lancet Neurology, 6,* 903–912.

Namey, M. A. (2011). Addressing risk factors across the disease spectrum. In C. Harris (Ed.), *Comprehensive nursing care in multiple sclerosis* (3rd ed., pp. 109–122). New York, NY: Springer Publishing Company.

O'Connor, P., Schwid, S. R., Herrmann, D. N., Markman, J. D., & Dworkin, R. H. (2008). Pain associated with multiple sclerosis: Systematic review and proposed classification. *Pain, 137,* 96–111.

Rizzo, M. A., Hadjimichael, O. C., Preiningerova, J., & Vollmer, T. L. (2004). Prevalence and treatment of spasticity reported by multiple sclerosis patients. *Multiple Sclerosis, 10,* 589–595.

Srivastava, A., Gupta, A., Taly, A. B., & Murali, T. (2009). Surgical management of pressure ulcers during inpatient neurologic rehabilitation: Outcomes for patients with spinal cord disease. *Journal of Spinal Cord Medicine, 32*(2), 125.

16

Pain and Multiple Sclerosis

OBJECTIVES

Upon completion of this chapter, the learner will be able to:

- Describe various pain syndromes in multiple sclerosis (MS)
- List medications used in the treatment of MS
- Describe nonpharmacologic strategies for pain management and MS
- Understand the impact of pain on individuals with MS

Pain is a significant symptom in multiple sclerosis (MS), and individuals with MS often rate pain as one of their most disabling symptoms. Chronic pain can lead to adverse disease outcomes, including impaired quality of life, depression, and loss of employment. The complexities of MS pain can result in the inadequate and inappropriate management of this symptom by health professionals. The nurse is in an ideal position to help patients develop an effective and individualized treatment plan.

- MS pain
  A. MS pain is complex.
  B. MS pain is a sensory phenomenon.
  C. MS pain is not adequately defined, identified, or measured by an observer.
  D. MS pain is an individualistic, learned, social, and cultural response.

- Proposed direct causes of MS pain
  A. Ephaptic transmission—short circuit between nerve fibers in areas of demyelination (e.g., trigeminal neuralgia)
  B. Inflammation around pain-sensitive structures (e.g., optic neuritis)
  C. Damage to the pain pathways in the central nervous system
  D. Sensitization of pain pathways leading to chronic neuronal hyperexcitability

- Other causes of pain in MS
  A. Pain may arise from other medical conditions (e.g., migraine, mechanical low back pain, fibromyalgia, arthritis).
  B. Musculoskeletal pain may occur as an indirect effect of MS due to stresses from spasticity, weakness, and deconditioning.

- Classifying MS pain
  A. Pain in MS is described by onset and duration—acute or chronic
    1. Acute syndromes—resolution over time
      a. Neuralgic pain (trigeminal neuralgia)
      b. Optic neuritis and retrobulbar pain
      c. Painful Lhermitte's syndrome
      d. Tonic spasms
    2. Chronic syndromes—ongoing and fluctuating
      a. Neurogenic pain (dysesthesia)
      b. Band-like pain in torso or extremities
      c. Musculoskeletal pain (low back pain)
      d. Spasticity/spasms

- Nature of pain—patient descriptors of MS pain (Melzack, 1987)
  A. Flickering, quivering, pulsing, throbbing, beating
  B. Pinching, pressing, gnawing, cramping
  C. Dull, sore, hurting, aching, heavy
  D. Spreading, radiating, penetrating, piercing
  E. Hot, burning, scalding, searing
  F. Tingling, itchy, smarting, stinging

- Approaching MS pain—factors to consider
  A. Date/time of occurrence of pain
  B. Location of pain

C. Description of pain (descriptors from the McGill Inventory, e.g., aching, prickly, burning)

D. Severity of pain—use simple visual analog scale from 0, being no pain, to 10, the worst pain ever

E. Strategies that have been used to manage pain including over-the-counter medications, complementary therapies, and prescription medications

F. Other contributing medical conditions

G. Relationship of pain to an acute MS relapse

H. Effect of depression and anxiety on pain

I. Factors that improve or worsen the pain (time of day, activities, heat/cold, certain positions)

J. Other new symptoms (especially for acute pain)

- The impact of MS pain
  A. Depression
  B. Anxiety
  C. Hopelessness
  D. Addiction and tolerance fears
  E. Sleeplessness
  F. Work and relationship loss
  G. Suicidal ideation

- Managing MS pain
  A. Educate patient and family about pain
  B. Encourage realistic goals
  C. Address factors that might exacerbate pain (while also treating the pain): anxiety, depression, sleeplessness, psychosocial stressors, inactivity
  D. Explore nonpharmacologic strategies
  E. Direct patient toward medications tailored to the nature and severity of the pain (balance relief of pain with side effects)

- Nonpharmacologic treatment
  A. Exercise—conditioning, stretching, yoga
  B. Physiotherapy—helps pain related to musculoskeletal conditions, spasticity, and muscle weakness
  C. Acupuncture
  D. Yoga

    E. Biofeedback

    F. Other—warmth, cold, relaxation, humor, distraction (Bowling, 2014)

■ Complexities of MS pain management often require a team approach

    A. Rehabilitation specialists—physio therapy, occupational therapy

    B. Psychologist—imagery, hypnosis

    C. Pain specialists—pain clinics

    D. Palliative care clinicians

    E. Recreational specialists

    F. Complementary therapy specialists

■ Monitor pain management outcomes

    A. Instruct the patient to:

        1. Keep a diary of the individual pain

        2. Use a visual analog scale to measure intensity

        3. Note time and magnitude of response—use visual analog scale again

        4. Make notation of treatment side effects

        5. Let clinicians know about satisfaction/dissatisfaction with pain management strategies

Table 16.1 Pharmacologic Management of Pain

Drug	Dose	Adverse effect
Gabapentin (Neurontin)	100–3,000 mg/d	Fatigue, somnolence
Carbamazepine (Tegretol)	400–800 mg/ bid	Dizziness, drowsiness
Pregabalin (Lyrica)	25 mg–300 mg/day	Dizziness, GI sx, weight gain, edema
Amitriptyline (Elavil)	10–150 mg/d	Drowsiness, dry mouth
Topiramate (Topamax)	25–400 mg/d	Fatigue, somnolence, cognitive impairment
Oxcarbazepine (Trileptal)	150–1,200 mg/d	Dizziness, somnolence
Duloxetine (Cymbalta)	30 mg–120 mg/d	GI sx, fatigue, dizziness

bid, twice a day; GI, gastrointestinal; sx, symptoms.

TABLE 16.2 Management Based on Assessment

What patient may feel	Type of pain	Treatment
Chronic burning, tingling, tightness, dull ache; often worse at night, after exercise, with warm temperature	Dysesthetic pain	Tricyclic antidepressants (amitriptyline), gabapentin, other anticonvulsants, sativex cannabinoid spray
Intense episodic painful burning, aching, itching of body, or, most often, the legs	Paroxysmal limb pain	Tricyclic antidepressants (e.g., amitriptyline), gabapentin, other anticonvulsants, sativex cannabinoid spray; heat/cold application
Aching caused by physical immobility	Musculoskeletal pain	Stretching; posture and gait evaluation; exercise; nonsteroidal anti-inflammatory agents (e.g., ibuprofen); proper seating; position changes; application of heat/cold
Pain travelling down the face, usually on just one side. Excruciating, sharp, shock-like.	Trigeminal neuralgia	Medication: carbamazepine, gabapentin, phenytoin, other anticonvulsants, baclofen, misoprostol
Pain in the eye, worse with eye movement	Optic neuritis	Corticosteroids, nonsteroidal anti-inflammatory agents (e.g., ibuprofen)
Brief muscle twitching or sudden sharp muscle spasm in the arm or leg; can occur a number of times throughout the day	Tonic spasms	Carbamazepine, gabapentin, other anticonvulsants
Muscle cramping, pulling, pain, and tightness	Spasms and spasticity	Stretching exercises; medications such as baclofen, tizanidine, botox (focal), dantrolene

(*continued*)

TABLE 16.2 Management Based on Assessment (*continued*)

What patient may feel	Type of pain	Treatment
Pain associated with pressure sores; bladder retention/infection; joint stiffness or contracture	Secondary pain of MS symptoms	Treatment of the underlying cause usually alleviates pain
Migraine, tension-type headache, cluster headache	Headache	Treatment determined by type of headache
Pain caused by MS therapies, such as flulike symptoms, headache, injection site reactions, and osteoporosis	Iatrogenic pain	Determined by patient's doctor and nurse, plus prevention
MS, multiple sclerosis.		

SUMMARY

■ Patients experiencing MS pain should

A. Identify the type of pain experience

B. Feel that their health care provider views their pain experience as real

C. Reduce their pain through behavioral strategies, rehabilitation, medications, or complementary therapies

D. Adopt coping strategies

E. Exhibit improved participation in usual daily activities

RESOURCES

Bowling, A. (2014). Optimal health with multiple sclerosis. In *A Guide to integrating lifestyle, alternative therapies, and conventional medicine*. New York, NY: Demos Medical.

Foley, P. L., Vesterinen, H. M., Laird, B. J., Sena, E. S., Colvin, L. A., Chandran, S., . . . Fallon, M. T. (2012). Prevalence and natural history of pain in adults with multiple sclerosis: Systematic review and meta-analysis. *Pain, 154*, 632–642.

Jawahar, R., Unsong, O., Yang, S., & Lapane, K. L. (2013). A systemic review of pharmacological pain management in multiple sclerosis. *Drugs, 73*, 1711–1722.

Melzack, R. (1975). The McGill Pain Questionnaire: Major properties and scoring methods. *Pain, 1*(3), 277–299.

Melzack, R. (1987). The short-form McGill Pain Questionnaire. *Pain, 30*(2), 191–197.

Shahrbanian, S., Auais, M., Duquette, P., Anderson K., & Mayo, N. E. (2013). Does pain in individuals with multiple sclerosis affect employment? *Pain Research and Management, 18*(5), e94–e100.

Truni, A., Barbanti, P., Pozzilli, C., & Cruccu, G. (2013). A mechanism-based classification of pain in multiple sclerosis. *Journal of Neurology, 260*(2), 1–20.

V

Functional Alterations: Personal Domain

17

Psychosocial Implications of Multiple Sclerosis

OBJECTIVES

Upon completion of this chapter, the learner will be able to:

- *Describe initial and ongoing emotional reactions to the diagnosis of multiple sclerosis (MS)*
- *Discuss the psychosocial impact of worsening disease*
- *Identify the environmental, financial, and ethnocultural implications of MS*
- *Cite therapeutic nursing interventions in support of patients and their families*

- Reactions to the diagnosis will evolve as the person with multiple sclerosis (MS) learns to cope with the ever-present reality of the disease:
    A. Shock
    B. Disbelief
    C. Denial
    D. Anger
    E. Depression
    F. Despair

G. Curiosity

H. Information seeking

I. Needing to affiliate with others

J. Wanting to be cured

K. Facing the reality of change

L. Confronting the impact of a chronic and sometimes disabling illness

M. Constant need for contact with the health care community

N. Navigating the world of insurance, reimbursement, and finances

■ Unique issues specific to MS

A. There is a greater understanding of MS with an emphasis on early intervention, although symptomatic management and emotional support remain mainstays of treatment.

1. Rehabilitation services are of great value throughout the disease spectrum.

2. Counseling, education, and advocacy are important roles for the nursing professional.

B. People with MS are faced with having to adapt to unpredictable change.

C. There are issues of abuse and neglect, divorce and separation, and altered body image, along with cultural, educational, and language variability.

D. We now know that MS can result in a high level of depression throughout a lifetime with the disease.

1. Treatment of depression may include pharmacologic and nonpharmacologic interventions.

E. Cognitive issues and other invisible symptoms can cause anxiety and fear in all those affected by MS.

1. Assessment is critical to identify problems.

2. Newer rehabilitation strategies may be beneficial and are now being investigated.

F. The challenge is to sustain a high level of support throughout a lifetime with the disease.

G. Strategies may include pharmacologic management, counseling, education, and ongoing mobilization of resources.

■ Informational needs of MS nursing professionals

A. Ethnocultural sensitivity

B. Gender-specific information

  C. Need to assess family resources
  D. Need for environmental adaptations
  E. Need for life planning

- Impact on future relationships
- Need for advocacy to access programs and services
- Sustaining realistic hope
- Employment issues:
  A. Reasonable accommodations
  B. Vocational rehabilitation
  C. Telecommuting
  D. Cognitive implications
  E. Educational concerns

- Impact on the family
  A. Alterations in roles and responsibilities
  B. Family planning, childbearing, and child-rearing concerns
  C. Changing lifestyles and economic circumstances
  D. Grief work balanced with hope

- How information helps children
  A. Provides reassurance
  B. Allays fears
  C. Gives them a vocabulary
  D. Reduces secrecy
  E. Promotes trust
  F. Gives symptoms a name

- Managing change in MS
  A. Education about the disease throughout a lifetime
  B. Counseling and support groups
  C. Crisis intervention
  D. Long-term planning/life planning
  E. Being flexible
  F. Finding hope
  G. Seeking wellness
  H. Using appropriate resources

RESOURCES

Amato, M. P. (2012). Cognitive and psychosocial issues in pediatric multiple sclerosis: Where we are and where we need to go. *Neuropediatrics, 43*(4), 174–175.

Borreani, C., Gianchi, E., Pietrolongo, E. Rossi, I., Cilia, S., Giuntoli, M., . . . PeNSAMI project. (2014). Unmet needs of people with severe multiple sclerosis and their carers: Qualitative findings for a home-based intervention. *PLoS One, 9*(10), e109679.

Grose, J., Freeman, J., & Skirton, H. (2012, Fall). Value of a confidant relationship in psychosocial care of people with multiple sclerosis. *International Journal of MS Care, 214*(3), 115–122.

Halper, J. (Ed.). (2007). *Advanced concepts in multiple sclerosis nursing care.* New York, NY: Demos Medical.

Halper, J., & Holland, N. (2011). Education of the patient and family. In J. Halper & N. Holland (Eds.), *Comprehensive nursing care in multiple sclerosis* (3rd ed., pp. 29–42). New York, NY: Springer Publishing Company.

Holland, N. J., & Halper, J. (2005). *Staying well with multiple sclerosis: A self-care guide.* New York, NY: Demos Medical.

Jobin, C., Larochelle, C., Parpal, H., Coyle, P. K., & Duquette, P. (2010). Gender issues in multiple sclerosis: An update. *Womens Health (London England), 6*(6), 797–820.

Kalb, R. C. (2011). Acknowledging sexuality and implementing family planning. In J. Halper & N. Holland (Eds.), *Comprehensive nursing care in multiple sclerosis* (pp. 169–192). New York, NY: Springer Publishing Company.

Kalina, J. T. (2014, Fall). Clutter management for individuals with multiple sclerosis. *International Journal of MS Care, 15*(3), 117–122.

Khan, F., Ng, L., & Turner-Stokes, L. (2009). Effectiveness of vocational rehabilitation intervention on the return to work and employment of persons with multiple sclerosis. *Cochrane Database of Systematic Reviews, 91*, CD007256.

Kouzoupis, A. B., Paparrigopoulos, T., Soldatos, M., & Papadimitriou, G. N. (2010). The family of the multiple sclerosis patient: A psychosocial perspective. *International Review of Psychiatry, 22*(1), 83–89.

La Rocca, N., & Kalb, R. C. (2006). *Multiple sclerosis: Understanding cognitive challenges.* New York, NY: Demos Medical.

La Rocca, N. G., & Kalb, R. C. (2011). Addressing psychosocial issues. In J. Halper & N. Holland (Eds.), *Comprehensive nursing care in multiple sclerosis* (pp. 131–168). New York, NY: Springer Publishing Company.

Rog, D., Burgess, M., Mottershead, J., & Talbot, P. (2010). *Multiple sclerosis answers at your fingertips.* London, UK: Class.

18

Financial and Vocational Concerns

OBJECTIVES

Upon completion of this chapter, the learner will be able to:

- Discuss the variability of insurance coverage in multiple sclerosis (MS) and other chronic conditions
- Describe factors that promote and hinder employment of persons with MS
- Describe vocational rehabilitation assistance programs

- Cost of living with multiple sclerosis (MS)
  - A. Reasons for determining costs include:
    1. Guide the selection of treatment modalities
    2. Guide the allocation of research dollars
    3. Locate hidden costs
  - B. Costs of MS over a lifetime vary from country to country; they may result from lost wages, medical costs, and inestimable family expenses.
  - C. Quality-of-life issues have inestimable value to patients and families as life changes in response to relapsing and progressive forms of the disease.

- Health insurance programs
  - A. U.S. private health insurance plans
    1. Traditional indemnity plan
    2. Managed care plans
    3. Health maintenance organizations
    4. Preferred provider organizations
    5. Affordable Care Act option in conjunction with government, private carriers, and Medicaid
  - B. U.S. governmental plans
    1. Supplemental Security Income
    2. Social Security Disability
    3. Civilian Health and Medical Program of the Department of Veterans Affairs (VA)
    4. Medicare
    5. Medicaid
  - C. Canadian health care system
    1. All people receive health care coverage
    2. Most people with MS must be assessed by MS specialists for disease-modifying agents (not in all provinces)
    3. Some individuals have private insurance plans
  - D. Canadian governmental disability plans
    1. Canadian Pension Plan Disability Program

- Importance of employment
  - A. Promotes feelings of personal worth and self-esteem
  - B. Contributes to one's identity
  - C. Source of respect from others
  - D. Provides monetary income
  - E. Frequent source of health insurance

- Factors that influence unemployment
  - A. Demographics
    1. Age
    2. Education
    3. Female sex
    4. Laborer status (90% have a work history; 60% are working at the time of diagnosis)

B. Psychosocial
   1. Cognition
      a. Attention and concentration
      b. Memory, lack of ability to find stored information
      c. Visual–spatial deficits
      d. Executive function
      e. Limitations in work and social activities are correlated; the extent of cognitive decline is independent of the degree of physical disability
   2. Depression
   3. Motivation
   4. Denial of disability
   5. Limitations in work and social activities are correlated with the extent of cognitive decline independent of degree of physical disability
C. Physical
   1. Fatigue
   2. Gait and mobility
   3. Visual disturbance
   4. Bladder/bowel function
   5. Pain
   6. Heat sensitivity
   7. Variable course of disease
   8. Spasticity
D. Environment
   1. Accessibility
   2. High temperature
   3. Transportation

- Factors that enhance employment and work
  A. Level of education
  B. Psychological and social services
  C. Available vocational services

- Employment protection
  A. The Americans with Disabilities Act
     1. Prohibits discrimination on the basis of disability

2. Requires reasonable accommodation

3. Public transportation running on fixed schedules must accommodate the disabled person

B. Canada

1. There is a duty to accommodate disabled people in most provinces.

2. Public transportation must accommodate disabled people who work.

■ Vocational rehabilitation interventions

A. Social Security Administration in the United States

1. Put individuals in touch with agencies for:

a. Job counseling

b. Job training

c. Job placement

B. Rehabilitation programs/services

1. Ticket to Work and Work Incentive Improvement Act of 1999

C. Vocational rehabilitation agencies

1. Application

2. Eligibility

3. Joint program planning with rehabilitation counselor

4. Types of vocational rehabilitation services

D. Work incentive programs via using trial work periods without losing benefits

■ Summary

A. MS care is extremely costly, as is the cost of the illness over a lifetime.

B. Adjustments are required to promote continued employment.

C. Disease-modifying therapy, although costly, may result in sustained employment over a lifetime with MS.

D. The goal is to promote independent living with MS with a desired quality of life.

E. Cognition issues and fatigue are major barriers to employment.

RESOURCES

Burks, J. S., & Johnson, K. P. (Eds.). (2000). *Multiple sclerosis: Diagnosis, treatment, and rehabilitation*. New York, NY: Demos Medical.

Freaser, Q., Clemmons, D., & Bennett, F. (2002). *Multiple sclerosis: Psychosocial and vocational interventions.* New York, NY: Demos Medical.

Northrop, D. (2011). Providing advocacy for the patient with multiple sclerosis. In J. Halper & N. Holland (Eds.), *Comprehensive nursing care in multiple sclerosis* (3rd ed., pp. 43–52). New York, NY: Springer Publishing Company.

Northrop, D., Cooper, S. E., & Calder, K. (2007). *Health insurance resource manual. A guide for people with chronic disease and disability.* New York, NY: Demos Medical.

VI

*Shaping Multiple Sclerosis
Nursing Practice*

19

Special Needs in Multiple Sclerosis

OBJECTIVES

Upon completion of this chapter, the learner will be able to:

- Describe the importance of the maintenance of a balanced health state
- Discuss primary care needs in multiple sclerosis (MS)
- Cite specific wellness activities in MS for men and women
- Describe characteristics and nursing implications in pediatric MS
- Assess special issues seen in the aging population with MS

- Regular physical examinations are essential for men and women with multiple sclerosis (MS). They should include the following:

    A. Blood work (complete blood count [CBC], comprehensive profile, and thyroid function tests)

    B. Height and weight if possible

    C. Blood pressure

    D. Assessment for risk factors (osteoporosis, diabetes, etc.)

    E. Education regarding exercise, smoking, diet, etc.

    F. Appropriate screenings and immunizations

G. Screening diagnostic investigations

1. CBC

2. Metabolic blood profile

3. Electrocardiograms at appropriate ages

4. Prostate-specific antigen for men older than 50 years

5. Pap smears and mammography examinations per gynecologic protocol

■ Hormonally mediated events

A. Pregnancy (there is a 70% reduction in risk of exacerbation during pregnancy and a 70% increase 3–6 months postpartum)

1. Education should include assessment of:

a. The patient's capabilities before conception

i. Cessation of medications prior to conception after consultation with neurologist and obstetrician/gynecologist

b. Available supports for the postpartum period

c. Considerations regarding breastfeeding versus bottle-feeding, issues of fatigue, disease-modifying agents

d. The family's living situation and economic resources

2. Menstrual cycle assessment should include normal cycle, premenstrual syndrome, cramping, bloating, and current medications.

a. Steroids, disease-modifying therapies (interferons, mitoxantrone, and cyclophosphamide) can cause menstrual irregularities.

3. Menopause—a paucity of research exists in this area. Current information about hormone replacement therapy (HRT) is confusing regarding risk reduction for osteoporosis and for coronary heart disease and osteoporosis. However, cancer and venous thromboembolism risks of long-term HRT are a current concern for many women. Menopausal hormone therapy has a complex pattern of risks and benefits, so consultation with a gynecologist may be recommended.

■ Recognizing and preventing pseudoexacerbations should include the following caveats:

A. Avoid increasing core body temperature (fever).

B. Maintain body core temperature with cooling devices, cool drinks, and cool showers if ambient temperature is high.

C. Cool down frequently when exercising (fan, cold drink, and light clothing), and exercise in a cool environment.

D. Treat infections promptly.

■ Osteoporosis

A. May occur in both men and women with MS

B. Is associated with reduced mobility and use of corticosteroids

C. Falls may result in fractures and increased disability

D. Assessment should include bone density study (DXA); a z-score of less than −2.0 requires treatment

E. Treatment consists of:

1. Education about risk reduction and safety measures at home

2. Exercise recommended for the prevention and treatment of osteoporosis

3. Lifestyle modifications such as smoking cessation and decreased alcohol and caffeine intake

4. Protective pads should be worn around the outer thigh covering the trochanteric region of the hip

5. Optimal calcium (1,000–1,500 mg/d) intake with vitamin D (400 IU for those younger than 65 years; 600–800 IU for those who are older)

6. Vitamin D is under investigation for optimal dose and blood levels

7. Estrogen therapy is controversial at this time (results of the Women's Health Initiative)

8. Selectic estrogen receptor modultors (SERMs; raloxifene or tamoxifen) may have potential benefit

9. Bisphosphonates are the drugs of choice

   a. Alendronate (daily or weekly)

   b. Risedronate

   c. Ibandronate sodium monthly

   d. Reclast or zoedronic acid annually

10. Research studies evaluating effect of:

    a. Calcitonin

    b. Parathyroid hormone

11. Preventing bone loss and vertebral fractures can be attained to some degree with any of the currently approved medications, exercise, and possibly diet. A person who has sustained a fracture is certainly a candidate for pharmacologic therapy.

■ Pulmonary complications

A. Pulmonary dysfunction secondary to MS is a leading cause of morbidity and mortality in MS.

   B. Assessment should include history of pneumonia, aspiration, dyspnea, weak cough, hypophonia, and fatigue.

   C. Treatment is predicated on noninvasive interventions whose goals are to

      1. Prevent respiratory failure

      2. Maintain normal lung ventilation

      3. Maintain normal lung compliance

      4. Help eliminate airway secretions through more effective cough flow

      5. Avoid upper respiratory infections, particularly during the influenza season

■ **Pediatric MS**

   A. Not as readily diagnosed as in adult population

   B. May present with systemic illness

      1. Fever

      2. Listlessness

   C. Less likely to have immunologic changes in cerebrospinal fluid

   D. Diagnostic markers may be different in children

   E. Other conditions must be ruled out during the diagnostic period

      1. Acute disseminated encephalomyelitis

      2. Mitochondrial disorders

      3. Lymphoma

      4. Leukodystrophies

      5. Vasculopathies

   F. There are treatment challenges based on age, developmental stage, and level of family understanding and support

      1. Disease modification

      2. Treatment of relapses

      3. Symptomatic management

      4. Psychosocial issues

         a. Feelings of indifference

         b. Stigma of chronic illness

         c. Need for:

            i. Informational support

            ii. Emotional support

            iii. Family involvement

RESOURCES

Boyd, J., & Milazzo, M. C. (2011). Working with the pediatric patient diagnosed with multiple sclerosis. In J. Halper & N. J. Holland (Eds.), *Comprehensive nursing care in multiple sclerosis* (3rd ed., pp. 193–214). New York, NY: Springer Publishing Company.

Coyle, P. K. (1998). Multiple sclerosis. In P. W. Kaplan (Ed.), *Neurologic disease in women* (pp. 251–264). New York, NY: Demos Medical.

Dobson, J., Kuhle, J., Baker, D., Giovannoni, G., & Ramagopalan, S. (2013). The effect of vitamin D-related interventions on multiple sclerosis relapses: A meta-analysis. *Multiple Sclerosis, 19*(12), 1571–1579.

Halper, J. (2002). Women's issues in multiple sclerosis. In J. Halper (Ed.), *Advanced concepts in multiple sclerosis nursing care* (pp. 141–145). New York, NY: Demos Medical.

Halper, J. (2007). Optimal primary care for people with multiple sclerosis. In J. Halper (Ed.), *Advanced concepts in multiple sclerosis nursing care* (pp. 47–57). New York, NY: Demos Medical.

Hanley, D. A., Cranney, A., Johnes, G., Whiting, S. J., Leslie, W. D., Cole, D. E., . . . Guidelines Committee of the Scientific Advisory Council of Osteoporosis Canada. (2010). Vitamin D in adult health and disease: A review and guideline statement from Osteoporosis Canada. *Canadian Medical Association Journal, 182*, E610–E618.

Hill, E. (n.d.). *Vitamin D levels associated with frailty in women.* Retrieved from www.medscape.com/viewarticle/734355

Lehman, L., & Picone, M. A. (2007). Pulmonary complications. In J. Halper (Ed.), *Advanced concepts in multiple sclerosis nursing care* (pp. 137–148). New York, NY: Demos Medical.

Manson, J., Chlebowski, R., Rowan, T., Stefanick, M., Aragaki, A., Rossouw, J., . . . Wallace, R. B. (2013). Menopausal hormone therapy and health outcomes during intervention and extended poststopping phases of the Women's Health Initiative randomized trials. *JAMA, 310*(13), 1353–1368.

McGuire, K. B., Stojanovic-Radic, J., Chiaravalloti, N. D., & DeLuca, J. (2015, January–February). Development and effectiveness of a psychoeducational wellness program for people with multiple sclerosis: Description and outcomes. *International Journal of MS Care, 17*(1), 1–8.

Nieves, J. W., & Cosman, F. (2002, July). Management strategies for osteoporosis. *Emergency Medicine,* 37–48.

Stokowski, L. A. (n.d.). *Vitamin D in the older adult.* Retrieved from www.medscape.com/viewarticle/733968_print

20

The Nurse's Role in Multiple Sclerosis Research

OBJECTIVES

Upon completion of this chapter, the learner will be able to:

- Describe the roles and responsibilities of the nurse in multiple sclerosis (MS) research
- Identify key concepts in the research process

- Roles of the research coordinator
  - A. Liaison
  - B. Facilitator
  - C. Educator
  - D. Administrator
  - E. Recruiter
  - F. Advocate
    1. Protecting human rights
    2. Nurturing patient retention
    3. Maintaining regulatory files
    4. Providing accurate documentation
    5. Promoting adherence to the protocol

6. Clarifying false expectations

7. Recognizing and reporting adverse events

8. Inspiring hope

■ Study files notebook includes the following:

A. Protocol—all versions

B. Protocol amendments

C. Consent forms—all versions

D. Investigator's brochure

E. 1572 forms and all updates

F. Curricula vitae of all those listed in 1572

G. Institutional review board (IRB) approvals

H. IRB membership

I. IRB correspondence

J. Safety reports

K. Serious adverse event (SAE) reports

L. Laboratory documents (normal values and certificates)

M. Drug accountability log

N. Sponsor correspondence

O. Monitoring log

P. Enrollment log

■ Definition of terms

A. Protocol—a framework for the conduct of the study.

B. Investigator's brochure—a detailed, confidential description of the structure and formulation of the drug and a summary of the studies and adverse events.

C. Form 1572—the official document that secures the investigator's commitment to conduct the study within U.S. Food and Drug Administration guidelines.

D. Source documents—documents that contain all the clinical information gathered during a visit.

E. Case report forms—concise information reflective of the source documents entered into duplicate forms that are collected and returned to the sponsor for data entry.

■ Trial design

A. Open label—the investigators and patients are aware of what drug or treatment is being tested.

B. Single-blinded study—the patient is blinded to the treatment, but the investigator is aware of what is being tested.

C. Double-blinded study—neither the investigator nor the patient knows who has been randomly assigned to what treatment (active therapy or placebo).

D. Crossover study—participants receive either placebo or tested therapy over a specific time, then investigational drug for the remainder of the study.

- Trial phases

A. Phase 1—designed to determine the metabolism and pharmacologic actions of a drug on human subjects.

  1. Determines the side effects associated with increasing doses of drug.

  2. Gain early evidence as to the effectiveness of a drug.

  3. Enrolls 20 to 80 subjects; subjects are often volunteers.

B. Phase 2—well-controlled, closely monitored studies to evaluate the effectiveness of a drug for a particular indication.

  1. Determines the short-term side effects and risks of drug.

  2. Enrolls several hundred subjects, all with a diagnosis of the disease being studied.

C. Phase 3—expanded trials performed after preliminary evidence suggests that a drug may be effective.

  1. Intended to gather additional information regarding effectiveness and safety of the drug.

  2. Enrolls several hundred to thousands of subjects.

D. Phase 4—postmarketing studies.

  1. Designed to test an approved product on different groups.

  2. Needed if sponsor wishes a label change.

  3. Designed to look at issues that concern customers.

- The IRB determines that

A. Risks to subjects are minimized.

B. Risks to subjects are reasonable in relation to anticipated benefits.

C. Selection of subjects is equitable.

D. Informed consent is obtained from the subjects or from a legal representative.

E. The research has a rational scientific basis, as does the methodology.

F. The research plan makes adequate provision for monitoring the data to ensure the safety of subjects.

G. There are adequate provisions to protect the privacy of the subject.

- Informed consent is based on ethical principles of full disclosure and the right of self-determination. The consent must be easily understood by a lay person and must contain the following:

  A. A statement that the study involves research

  B. An explanation of the purpose of the research, the design of the study, and the procedures that are experimental

  C. A description of any foreseeable risks or discomforts including, for women who are able to have children, risks to childbearing or to the fetus

  D. A description of potential benefits

  E. A disclosure of appropriate alternative procedures or course of treatment, if any, that may be advantageous to the subject

  F. A statement describing the extent to which confidentiality of records will be maintained, including the fact that the U.S. Food and Drug Administration might inspect the records

  G. For research involving more than a minimal risk, an explanation as to whether compensation and medical treatments are available

  H. An explanation of who should be contacted for answers to pertinent questions about the research and the research subject's rights

  I. A statement that participation is voluntary, refusal to participate will not result in any penalty or loss of service to which the subject is otherwise entitled, and that the subject may withdraw at any time without penalty

- Adverse events

  A. Adverse drug experience—any unfavorable and unintended sign, symptom, or disease temporally associated with the use of investigational product

  B. Serious adverse drug experience—any experience that results in death, a life-threatening adverse event, inpatient hospitalization or prolongation of hospitalization, or a persistent or significant disability or incapacity related to the research

  C. Unexpected adverse drug experience—any adverse experience, the specificity or severity of which is not consistent with the current investigator's brochure

- Nursing assessment

  A. How realistic are the patient's expectations of what the drug under study will and will not do for MS?

  B. Does the person understand that there might be a chance of receiving a placebo (in placebo-controlled studies)?

C. Is the patient committed to the frequency of visits, testing requirements, and procedures outlined in the consent form and protocol?

D. How successful has the patient been in the past in terms of keeping appointments and adhering to treatments?

E. Does the patient lack adequate insurance for currently available treatments?

F. Is the patient experiencing a decline in functional status despite aggressive therapeutic interventions?

- Recommendations for research nurse coordinators

A. A study has a beginning, middle, and end; there will be closure.

B. Study work will satisfy a compulsive nature, if you have one.

C. Keep in touch with other nurse coordinators for support and information.

D. Take care of yourself; this is hard work.

E. Participate in the investigators' meeting; this is your opportunity to share experiences with others and with the sponsor.

F. Think of research questions you may want to incorporate into the study; sponsors are often interested in other research questions.

- Evaluating research for practice

A. Does the research design answer the research question?

B. Are the research problem and purpose clearly stated?

C. Is the sample size adequate to generalize to target population and avoid Type II error and biases?

D. Are measurements clearly described, including validity and reliability of instruments?

E. Are data collection methods clearly stated and conducted in a consistent and ethical manner?

F. Is data analysis appropriate to address the research question and hypothesis?

G. Is an interpretation/discussion of findings addressed for each question and hypothesis, and is it unbiased?

- Terminology

A. Type I and Type II errors

1. A Type I error occurs when a researcher rejects the null hypothesis when it is actually true.

2. A Type II error is acceptance of the null hypothesis when it is false.

B. Level of significance

   1. The degree or probability of making a Type I or a Type II error.

   2. Most commonly used levels are alpha of .05 or .01.

■ Relevance to practice

   A. Nurses have an increasing need to base their practice on evidence.

   B. Evaluating research studies promotes a valid practice model.

   C. Patient and family education are facilitated by interpretation of research findings to recipients of care.

RESOURCES

Brinkman-Denney, S. (2013). An international comparison of the clinical trials nurse role. *Nursing Management, 20*(8), 32–40.

Gulick, E. E. (2007). The role of research in nursing practice. In J. Halper (Ed.), *Advanced concepts in multiple sclerosis nursing care* (pp. 101–110). New York, NY: Demos Medical.

Knapp, R. G. (2000). *Basic statistics for nurses.* Clifton Park, NY: Delmar, Cengage Learning.

Lowden, D. (2010). Measuring outcomes. In K. Costello & J. Halper (Eds.), *Advanced practice nursing in multiple sclerosis: Advanced skills, advancing responsibilities* (pp. 26–29). Washington, DC: EME.

Morgante, L. (2007). Research coordinator: Another dimension of MS nursing. In J. Halper (Ed.), *Advanced concepts in multiple sclerosis nursing care* (pp. 111–126). New York, NY: Demos Medical.

Pick, A. (2013). Informed consent in clinical research. *Nursing Standard, 27*(49), 44–47.

21

Complementary and Alternative Therapies

OBJECTIVES:

Upon completion of this chapter, the learner will be able to:

- *Identify the types of available therapies that are believed to be helpful in chronic illness*
- *Discuss the potential benefit/risk profile of these agents to educate patients and families appropriately*
- *Describe nonpharmacologic measures defined as complementary and alternative medicine/therapies (CAM) to assist patients to select interventions safely and appropriately*

- Defining complementary and alternative medicine/therapies (CAM)
  - A. CAM is defined as the combination of products and therapies found outside the standard, conventional medical treatments found in hospitals.
  - B. Some medical schools have developed "Integrated Medicine" departments to educate physicians about these options.
  - C. Usage of CAM is becoming commonplace.
    1. Studies have found a high incidence throughout the world.
    2. Literature reviews have substantiated this finding.

D. Types of CAM reported were exercise, vitamins, herbal and mineral supplements, relaxation techniques, acupuncture, cannabis, and massage.

E. Symptoms reported in the literature for which CAM is used are pain, fatigue, spasticity, stress, anxiety, and depression.

F. The National Institutes of Health has established five types of CAM therapy:

1. Biologically based: diet and supplements

2. Mind–body: meditation, hypnosis, spirituality

3. Manipulative and body-based systems: massage, chiropractic

4. Alternative medical systems: Chinese medicine, Ayurveda

5. Energy therapies: magnets, therapeutic touch

■ How to work with patients who are using CAM

A. Ask routinely and in a nonjudgmental manner what CAMS are used (herbs, vitamins, supplements).

B. Explore the individual's reasons for wanting to use CAMS.

C. Suggest the incorporation of CAMS into proven conventional treatment if not contraindicated; if not advisable, educate the patients about risk/benefit profile.

D. Encourage patients to evaluate their response to CAMS on a regular basis.

E. Continue to provide accurate information about efficacy, safety, and cost.

F. Provide patients with information about resources.

■ Sources of information about CAM

A. Books

B. Journals and magazines

C. Peer support programs

D. Internet resources

E. Medical/professional resources

RESOURCES

Bowling, A. C. (2007). *Alternative medicine and multiple sclerosis.* New York, NY: Demos Medical.

Bowling, A. C. (2010). Unconventional medicine and multiple sclerosis: The role of conventional health providers. In C. F. Lucchinetti & R. Hohlfeld (Eds.), *Multiple sclerosis* (pp. 355–368). Philadelphia, PA: Saunders Elsevier.

Bowling, A. C. (2014). *Optimal health with multiple sclerosis: A guide to integrating lifestyle, alternative therapies, and conventional medicine.* New York, NY: Demos Medical.

Bowling, A. C., & Stewart, T. M. (2004). *Dietary supplements and multiple sclerosis.* New York, NY: Demos Medical.

Hooper, K. D., Pender, M. P., Webb, P. M., & McCombe, P. A. (2001). The use of traditional and complementary medical care by patients with multiple sclerosis in south-east Queensland. *International Journal of MS Care, 24,* 13–28.

Kennedy, P. (2007). Complementary and alternative therapies. In J. Halper (Ed.), *Advanced concepts in multiple sclerosis nursing care* (pp. 225–240). New York, NY: Demos Medical.

Lovera, J., Bagert, B., Smoot, K., Morris, C. D., Frank, R., Bogardus, K., . . . Bourdette, D. (2007). *Ginkgo biloba* for the improvement of cognitive performance in multiple sclerosis: A randomized, placebo-controlled trial. *Multiple Sclerosis, 13,* 376–385.

Polman, C. H., Thompson, A. J., Murray, T. J., & McDonald, W. I. (2006). *Multiple sclerosis: The guide to treatment and management* (pp. 117–179). New York, NY: Demos Medical.

Stewart, T. M., & Bowling, A. C. (2005). Polyunsaturated fatty acid supplementation in MS. *International Journal of MS Care, 12,* 88–93.

Yadav, V., Bever C., Jr., Bowling, A., Weinstock-Guttman, B., Cameron, M., . . . Narayanaswami, P. (2014). Summary of evidence based guidelines: Complementary and alternative medicine in multiple sclerosis. *Neurology, 82*(12), 1083–1092.

INTERNET RESOURCE

National Multiple Sclerosis Society: Complementary & Alternative Medicines (www.nationalmssociety.org/Treating-MS/Complementary-Alternative-Medicines)

Appendices

A

Overview: Case Studies

These case studies are to assist our readers to problem solve using real-life situations. They do not reflect the format of the multiple sclerosis (MS) certification examination, but are provided to promote critical thinking.

CASE STUDY 1

Sally is 34 years old and was diagnosed with MS in 2002. She initially experienced a relapsing–remitting course in which her exacerbations were mild and occurred infrequently. After her second pregnancy, about 6 months postpartum, she had a severe exacerbation that resulted in paralysis of both lower extremities. Following hospitalization for intravenous steroids, she was treated in an inpatient rehabilitation hospital for strengthening and improvement of function. When she was discharged, she was able to walk with a wheeled walker, and she used a motorized tricart for longer distances.

Over the past 3 years, her ability to walk has diminished. She is able to stand and pivot for transfers and take only a few steps to and from chairs and her bed. She continues to experience attacks of her MS, and despite treatment with steroids, she has had incomplete recovery. She now requires maximal assistance to get in and out of her car. She uses a tub transfer chair to bathe and grab bars to get up and down from her commode. She uses a long-handled reacher in her kitchen and bedroom to reach items on high shelves. She has had a ramp installed at her front door and has widened the doorways in her home to accommodate her scooter. She is subject to fatigue and finds that if she rests in the afternoons, she is able to stay up until 9:00 or 10:00 p.m. before going to bed.

Sally and her family have had frequent contact with the National Multiple Sclerosis Society, participating in several educational programs, family weekends, and support groups. Sally receives her care at an MS center where, in addition to neurologic care, she has had nursing care for bladder and bowel management, counseling to assist her to adjust to her changing physical condition, and rehabilitation services. She has had physical therapy for mobility and to develop a home program and for occupational therapy for upper extremity function and the appropriate use of assistive devices. Her current medications consist of oxybutynin for her bladder, modafinil for fatigue, and gabapentin for pain. Sally's condition continues to worsen, and her neurologist has discussed immunomodulating therapy, since her MRI and her history reveal that she continues to have relapses, but has not suggested a particular product. Sally is unsure about what to do and comes to you for advice and education.

Management Considerations

1. Factors to consider in assisting Sally with her decision regarding therapy.
   - Cost of therapy and her insurance coverage
   - Efficacy of the proposed treatment and tolerability
   - Her ability to manage the proposed therapy
   - Impact on her quality of life
2. Patient education required to assist Sally and her family once a decision is made to begin therapy.
   - Mechanisms of action of selected therapy
   - Long-term safety and potential adverse reactions
   - Managing side effects
   - What she can expect from therapy
   - Importance of adherence to medication and required laboratory monitoring
3. Strategies that have been shown to facilitate adherence to complex protocols:
   - A strong and trusting health provider/patient relationship
   - A supportive MS peer network
   - Education for informed decision making
   - Consideration of health literacy when therapeutic education is provided
4. Sally has occasional short-term memory problems, particularly when she is fatigued. Strategies that can be used to help her to overcome this deficit and facilitate adherence:
   - Give simple, structured instructions
   - Reinforce the material frequently
   - Involve care partners in the care
   - Provide written material

CASE STUDY 2

Susan, a 24-year-old woman with MS diagnosed 3 years ago, presents to your practice. She has been taking the disease-modifying therapy (DMT) glatiramer acetate for 2 years with an inconsistent routine of injections and minimal health care follow-up. She lives with her boyfriend, and they have a very active lifestyle. She works full time and has a busy social life, getting 3 to 4 hours of sleep each night and eating irregularly. Medications consist of DMT, over-the-counter headache medications, oral contraceptive, and modafinil 200 mg bid. She presents to the MS center complaining of nausea, vomiting, dizziness, and severe fatigue. Neurologic examination is negative except for a positive Romberg test. U/A via dipstick is positive for leukocyte esterase. Vital signs: BP 120/80; HR 100, lungs clear. Patient is afebrile. Her last menstrual period was 6 weeks ago.

Management Considerations

1. Issues to rule out immediately
   - Pregnancy
   - Urinary tract infection
   - Acute relapse versus pseudo relapse
   - Other health conditions
2. Health and wellness areas that should be discussed with Susan
   - Sleep hygiene
   - Diet, adequate fluid intake, and exercise
   - Importance of adherence to DMT and oral contraceptive
   - Smoking, drug and alcohol use
3. Education on medication use should include
   - Impact of modafinil and other medications on efficacy of oral contraceptives
   - Impact of excessive use of over-the-counter headache medications
   - Ensuring that daily adherence of glatiramer acetate is possible, and if not, considering other DMT options

CASE STUDY 3

William is a 35-year-old executive who works 50 to 60 hours/wk and travels frequently. He has a 7-year history of MS. Initially, he had infrequent exacerbations that were treated with short courses of either intravenous or oral steroids. Two years ago, he developed bilateral lower extremity weakness, a T10 sensory level, and forgetfulness. Treatment was begun with dimethyl fumarate, which he uses inconsistently because he does not see himself "getting better." He has difficulty remembering to take his second dose of the day, and is reluctant to ask his family for assistance with reminders. William has become increasingly anxious. His social situation and work have suffered, and he is becoming more isolated.

Management Considerations

1. The treatment approach for this patient should include:
   - Discussion of psychosocial concerns
   - Review of his treatment expectations
   - Counseling regarding energy conservation and vocational activities
   - Changing his DMT to an alternate therapy with consideration for efficacy and adherence ease
2. In addition, other services should be arranged for:
   - Vocational counseling and retraining
   - Physical therapy for exercise and gait training
   - Counseling for loss of physical abilities, altered lifestyle, and occupational difficulties
   - Discussion of long-term disability benefits
   - Family education and support

CASE STUDY 4

Kenneth is a 42-year-old man with a 10-year history of relapsing–remitting MS. He is no longer working, because of cognitive changes resulting from MS. He experienced two relapses during the past year, and both he and his wife are anxious to begin a disease-modifying agent as soon as possible. Kenneth is interested in initiating one of the injectable medications because he is comfortable with the long-term safety of these therapies. His wife has concerns about his ability to learn the injection technique.

Management Considerations

1. Educational strategies that will assist this couple in learning an injection procedure and potentially help minimize the concerns of the patient and his wife:
   - Audio and video material along with written instructions
   - Watching another patient self-inject
   - Demonstrating the technique to the nurse during one office visit
   - Having a visiting nurse teach the patient and wife at home

2. Adherence can be promoted by:
   - Calling the patient regularly after he begins self-injection
   - Asking that he keep records of his injection sites
   - Asking his wife to support his adherence
   - Referring him to a network of patients using the same medication
   - Scheduling a follow-up appointment in 2 to 3 months after starting injections

CASE STUDY 5

Maryann is a 27-year-old woman with a 3-year history of relapsing–remitting MS. She has had four relapses since her diagnosis and has recovered completely from all but the last relapse, which left her with sensory deficits in both feet. She works full time as a legal secretary and enjoys an active social life. Maryann is concerned about her incomplete recovery after her last relapse and wants to begin one of the new disease-modifying agents. Her neurologist presented her with all available treatment options, but felt that she should select the treatment that would best fit her lifestyle.

Management Considerations

1. Education about available treatments should be provided in a therapeutic environment and include:
   - Accurate information on mechanism of action, route of administration, and treatment schedule of all available therapies
   - Long-term risk and safety information
   - Expectations for pre- and posttreatment initiation laboratory monitoring and follow-up
   - Expectations of treatment effect and efficacy
2. All patient and family education in MS should:
   - Promote informed decision making
   - Empower patients to guide their own health care
   - Be evidence-based and provide objective information on efficacy and safety
   - Be delivered with consideration of culture and health literacy

CASE STUDY 6

Martin is a 23-year-old with a 5-year history of MS; he developed vertigo and incoordination of gait over a 7-day period, which stabilized and slowly improved over the next month. Two years later, the symptoms returned, along with ill-defined difficulty with blurred vision, which also improved when a course of high-dose steroids was given. Within the next year, he began to note severe spasticity of his lower extremities with resultant problems with gait, transfers, and bed mobility. Treatment with baclofen and tizanidine resulted in minimal improvement. His motor and cerebellar symptoms progressed, and he was nonambulatory at age 25. He was seen at the MS center complaining of pain and rigidity in his legs, bowel and bladder incontinence, and anxiety. He reported no cognitive difficulties. Martin is requesting treatment with immunomodulating therapy.

Management Considerations

1. Treatment priorities for this patient include:
   - Spasticity management
   - Counseling/education of appropriate management at this stage of his illness
   - Clarification of treatment goals as related to his quality of life
2. Additional interventions helpful to this patient at this time include:
   - Confirming that the patient understands his current health state
   - Evaluating and enhancing his support systems
   - Consideration of the initiation of a rehabilitation program

CASE STUDY 7

Felicia is 46 years old and has lived alone since her daughter went off to college. She has been divorced for 3 years, and has no other children or family who live close by. She has secondary-progressive MS and has minimal household assistance. She is fiercely independent, yet is exposed to household dangers (cooking, toileting, and bathing). She was hospitalized in August for an acute exacerbation (right-arm weakness and increased tremor), then sent to subacute rehabilitation. She made little progress and was advised that it would be safer for her to consider long-term living options (assisted living, nursing home) rather than return home. She refused and returned to her home, with 2 hours of home health aide assistance three times a week. She calls the MS center three or four times a week with questions and concerns. ("What medications am I on? I dropped my pills—I need more. I have no food in the house.") She still refuses to discuss living elsewhere.

Management Considerations

1. The primary concerns for this patient are:
   - Safety issues
   - Socialization concerns

- Emotional reaction to MS
- Isolation and loneliness

2. Therapeutic interventions for this patient should include:
   - Contacting the public health department in her town
   - Counseling the patient about dangers in her home
   - Continuing to support her in her decision with as much assistance as possible
   - Including her daughter in decision making where possible

3. Cognitive issues of concern in this situation include:
   - Impaired judgment
   - Poor executive function
   - Rigidity in personal care choices

4. Emotional reactions that an MS nurse might expect with this patient include:
   - Anger
   - Frustration
   - Hopelessness

CASE STUDY 8

Helen is a 46-year-old woman with a 25-year history of MS. She is wheelchair confined and has severe tremor. Her husband is a house painter and is away all day. Helen has two young children (12 and 10 years old) who are doing very poorly in school and who are not supervised in the afternoon. She sleeps a great deal during the day and is up most of the night. Her husband complains that he is unable to sleep and rest because of his wife's sleep patterns. She has emotional outbursts, screaming at her family for minimal infractions of "the rules," and is emotionally labile with unexpected crying jags. The children are having problems in school with homework, interpersonal relations, and cleanliness. The husband is overwhelmed and does not understand the problem. He feels his wife could do better if she tried.

Management Considerations

1. Education and information that could help this family at this time include:
   - Discussion of cognitive impairments and MS
   - Description of how MS has affected Helen
   - Exploring family members' understanding of and reactions to Helen's illness

2. Services that may be important to this family at this time include:
   - A home health aide for Helen

- A day program for Helen to provide social stimulation
- Assistance with the children when they return from school
3. Mental/social health services that might be helpful at this time include:
   - Neuropsychological evaluation
   - Psychiatric evaluation
   - Home health evaluation

CASE STUDY 9

Henry is a 28-year-old male with a 5-year history of active MS. He came to the reception desk of the MS center and reported a sudden onset of mild arm weakness and some subtle slurring of speech. He had been relapse free for the past 3 years since starting natalizumab. He is anti–JC virus positive and has previously been treated with interferon beta-1a and mitoxantrone. His only other medications are multivitamins and vitamin D. He was well informed of the risks of natalizumab use beyond 2 years in the presence of a positive anti–JC virus antibody status, but he has been able to enjoy his young son, and live an active normal life. His last natilizumab infusion was 3 weeks ago, and he has tolerated this medication very well. A recent urine culture is negative for an infection. On presentation, he was extremely anxious and tearful and informed the receptionist that the MS team are really going to want to see him.

Management Considerations

1. Concerns for this patient at this time include:
   - Acute MS relapse
   - Psychosocial crisis
   - Potential development of progressive multifocal leukoencephalopathy (PML)
2. Recommended treatment strategies include:
   - Notification of the patient's attending neurologist
   - Urgent MRI and LP
   - Rule out all other systemic infections
   - Discontinuation of natalizumab pending diagnostic workup

CASE STUDY 10

Gerald is a 42-year-old man with a 10-year history of MS. He is married, and has three children aged 14, 12, and 8 years. He served in the Navy before his marriage and then became a security guard at a local company. He has a gun collection in his home. He has brain stem symptoms (tremor, ataxia, and nystagmus) and is no longer able to work. He has been hospitalized three times during the past 5 years for paranoid behaviors, and after his most recent hospitalization, it was recommended by the care team that he remove the guns from his home. The guns, however, have not been removed. He has been tested for cognitive impairment (memory, judgment, and learning have been affected) and was counseled by a neuropsychologist until his insurance stopped covering the service.

Lately, he has become increasingly abusive to his wife and family. He threatens his wife and children with both physical abuse and with his guns. The children are having problems in school, and they are responsible for the patient's care when they return home in the afternoons. He is intermittently depressed and exhibits paranoid thoughts (e.g., his wife is having an affair, his daughter should have been aborted). Recently, his wife has been participating in counseling, but the patient refuses to do so. She has had to return to work because finances are a problem in light of the needs of the growing children. Gerald has told his home health aide that he plans to kill his wife.

Management Considerations

1. The role of the nurse upon hearing this information is to:
   - Report the situation to the charge nurse
   - Inform the patient's physician immediately
   - Contact the authorities
2. Provided the patient agrees to hospitalization, the following discharge planning would be necessary for this family:
   - Ongoing assessment and treatment by a mental health professional
   - Support groups for his wife and children
   - Day treatment program for the patient
   - Assurance of removal of guns
3. Other nursing interventions that would be helpful upon the patient's discharge include:
   - Patient and family education about the emotional aspects of MS
   - Advising the family to consider long-term placement if this situation continues to worsen
   - Ensuring that the home environment is safe for the patient and family

B

Personal Review Questions

1. Which of the following statements about the possible cause(s) of multiple sclerosis (MS) is incorrect?

    a. Abnormal autoimmune response to myelin develops after exposure to some environmental agent in genetically predisposed individuals

    b. Immune system activation

    c. Decreased production of inflammatory cytokines

    d. Combined effects of the autoimmune response cause the demyelination, axonal damage, and scarring seen in patients with MS

2. Onset of MS usually occurs in persons between the ages of:

    a. 20 to 30

    b. 40 to 50

    c. 10 to 30

    d. 30 to 50

3. According to the Poser Diagnostic Criteria, how many exacerbations, separated by at least 30 days, with neurologic symptoms referable to lesions in two different areas of white matter of the central nervous system (CNS) must a patient experience before a definite diagnosis of MS can be made?

    a. One

    b. Two

    c. Three

    d. Four

4. On onset, MS follows a relapsing–remitting pattern in approximately what percentage of patients?

    a. 50

    b. 85

    c. 30

    d. 15

5. Continuing care for a patient with relapsing–remitting MS does *not* include:

    a. Ensuring adequate access to medications and adaptive equipment

    b. Encouraging sustained treatment with a disease-modifying agent

    c. Discouraging patient autonomy

    d. Assisting patient and family with vocational issues

6. Sustaining care for patients with advanced MS may include:

    a. Interventions to prevent pressure sores

    b. Providing palliative care

    c. Discussing the value of wellness activities

    d. All of the above

7. Which of the following agents reduces relapse rates in MS?

    a. Lorazepam

    b. Prednisone

    c. Fingolimod

    d. Nortriptyline

8. A medication that may help reduce symptoms of fatigue is:

    a. Baclofen

    b. Amantidine

    c. Clonazepam

    d. Gabapentin

9. Disease-modifying therapies should be started early in the disease because they do all of the following except:

    a. Decrease relapse severity

    b. Reduce relapses

    c. Reverse MS symptoms

    d. Delay progression of disability

10. Which of the following complications is the leading cause of mortality in advanced MS?

    a. Fats

    b. Pneumosepsis

    c. Suicide

    d. Osteoporosis

11. As part of continuing care for patients with relapsing–remitting MS who have experienced a relapse, the nurse will need to:
    a. Recommend an immediate DMT switch
    b. Assess the patient's adherence to current DMT
    c. Advise the patient to take a drug holiday from the DMT
    d. Tell the patient not to be concerned at this time

12. Which of the following statements about the role of MS nurses is not correct?
    a. Cost-containment pressures brought about a dramatic and ongoing expansion in the role of the nurse.
    b. Advanced practice nurses have had decreasing prescriptive authority.
    c. The MS nurse provides primary, acute, specialized, and rehabilitative care for patients with multiple sclerosis.
    d. Nurses provide education, support, and health care delivery for patients and their families.

13. The aims of nursing research include all of the following except:
    a. Generating new knowledge
    b. Validating existing knowledge
    c. Guiding nursing practice
    d. Testing the efficacy of a new medication

14. Nurses who wish to conduct research can begin to seek funding and support by:
    a. Identifying funding sources
    b. Developing grant-writing skills
    c. Identifying and developing collaborative relationships
    d. All of the above

15. Which of the following statements about MS is correct?
    a. Life expectancy from time of diagnosis is generally 10 years.
    b. The age of onset is usually 40 to 60 years.
    c. MS affects more women than men.
    d. The recent development of a cure for MS has brought hope to patients and their families.

16. Which of the following statements about the pathophysiology of MS is true?
    a. The lesions associated with MS are particularly prevalent in the optic nerves and the gray matter of the spinal cord, brain stem, cerebellum, and cerebrum.
    b. Loss of the myelin sheath disrupts electrical conduction within the CNS.

    c. MS is thought to occur secondary to a bacterial infection.

    d. Myelin loss occurs only in the spinal cords of people with MS.

17. Which of the following statements about MS is not true?

    a. People with MS may experience neurologic deficits such as tremor, sensory loss, and bladder incontinence.

    b. Secondary symptoms of MS include bladder infections and pressure sores.

    c. Cognitive impairment in people with MS occurs rarely.

    d. Neurologic signs and symptoms associated with MS are dependent on the location of the lesions in the CNS.

18. Which of the following statements about MS is correct?

    a. MRI is the gold standard used to definitely diagnose MS.

    b. Evoked potential testing is not helpful in the diagnosis of MS.

    c. In approximately 85% of people with MS, the course is described as relapsing–remitting at the time of diagnosis.

    d. The course of MS is invariably characterized by progressive deterioration.

19. Which of the following statements is not true?

    a. PML is a potentially fatal brain infection that can occur with the use of natalizumab.

    b. Interferon beta-lb is an immunomodulating agent.

    c. Glatiramer acetate's mode of action involves inhibition of the immune response to myelin basic protein and other myelin antigens.

    d. Interferon beta-la is only administered intramuscularly.

20. Which of the following statements is correct?

    a. Adherence to medications requires information and support.

    b. Information should imply that there is no real risk associated with MS with or without treatment.

    c. Health care professionals should always be in charge of making decisions about treatment.

    d. People who think that their disease is not under their control adhere more readily to treatment.

21. You are caring for a patient with relapsing–remitting MS who has just started treatment with interferon therapy. Which information is least likely to facilitate adherence?

    a. Interferon reduces the frequency of exacerbations, but does not restore function.

    b. Interferon therapy has no side effects.

    c. Interferon is administered by injection only.

    d. Patients are encouraged to self-administer interferons.

22. Which of the following is not generally considered a barrier to adherence?

    a. Lack of knowledge

    b. Overly optimistic expectations

    c. Lack of financial support

    d. Age

23. Which of the following statements is not correct?

    a. Patient satisfaction has no effect on adherence.

    b. Empathizing with patients facilitates adherence.

    c. Cultural differences can influence adherence.

    d. Problems with reasoning can interfere with adherence.

24. Which of the following statements is incorrect?

    a. The severity of cognitive impairment varies from patient to patient.

    b. Many people with MS stop work early because of cognitive impairments.

    c. Cognitive impairment affects more than 95% of persons with MS.

    d. Relatively mild and subtle cognitive deficits may have an impact on patients' lives.

25. Which of the following cognitive functions is least likely to be affected in people with MS?

    a. Recall memory

    b. Long-term memory

    c. Information processing

    d. Attention and concentration

26. Which of the following statements is correct?

    a. The prevalence of MS-related cognitive impairment is estimated to be less than 20%.

    b. Studies using sensitive neuropsychologic instruments suggest that approximately half of the MS population experiences cognitive dysfunction.

    c. Until recently, the prevalence of cognitive impairment in people with MS was overestimated.

    d. Studies using sensitive neuropsychologic instruments suggest that approximately 80% of the MS population experiences cognitive dysfunction.

27. Which of the following statements is correct?

    a. People with minimal sensory and motor impairment are not at risk of cognitive impairment.

    b. A high correlation between the extent of cognitive impairment and indices of disability has not been demonstrated.

    c. Cognitive and neurologic deficits develop in parallel.

    d. There is a strong positive correlation between disease course and the development of cognitive impairment.

28. In which of the following scenarios is neuropsychologic evaluation not indicated?

    a. An employer reports that a patient is not working as productively as he had been.

    b. A baseline assessment of cognitive function is desired prior to initiating immunomodulating therapy.

    c. A family is concerned that a patient may have cognitive impairment, but the patient denies any problems, and there is no clinical evidence for such impairment.

    d. The patient reports cognitive deficits that, although subtle or fluctuating, may have functional impact.

29. Which of the following strategies is unlikely to help patients with severe cognitive deficits?

    a. Insight-oriented psychotherapy

    b. Family counseling

    c. Audiotaping information

    d. Minimizing distractions

30. Which of the following is the best approach that nurses can adopt when addressing quality-of-life issues with people who have MS?

    a. Nurses should encourage patients to aim for a higher quality of life.

    b. Nurses should recognize that each patient may have different expectations and aspirations.

    c. Nurses should constantly reevaluate the patient's quality of life.

    d. It is important to use quality-of-life questionnaires before initiating conversations about quality of life.

31. Which of the following statements is correct?

    a. The degree of disability is the sole determinant of quality of life in MS.

    b. Recognizing the need to respond to change is more important than the ability to socialize in MS.

   c. Impaired cognition does not affect quality of life.

   d. Developing and sustaining satisfying relationships is an important factor in MS.

32. In general terms, which of the following would be least likely to influence a person's quality of life in MS?

   a. Cognitive deficits

   b. Difficulty walking

   c. Numbness

   d. Family strain

33. The symptoms of multiple sclerosis result from:

   a. Inadequate lymphocyte production

   b. Proliferation of myelin

   c. Inadequate inflammatory response

   d. Demyelination and scarring of nerve fibers

34. Which of the following statements describes the process termed "molecular mimicry?"

   a. The immune system fails to react to a foreign substance.

   b. Lymphocytes release antibodies in response to an antigen.

   c. The foreign target and the self-target of the immune system share molecular features.

   d. An inflammatory process upregulates adhesion molecules on endothelial cells.

35. A patient asks about the purpose of a lumbar puncture. Which of these responses do you make?

   a. Analysis of cerebrospinal fluid is helpful when the results of other tests are inconclusive.

   b. If your cerebrospinal fluid is negative, it will confirm that you do not have MS.

   c. Examining your cerebrospinal fluid will help us predict the course of your disease.

   d. A positive result from the cerebrospinal fluid is a definitive test for MS.

36. Which of the following patients has the most favorable prognosis?

   a. 32-year-old woman with ataxia and dysarthria

   b. 28-year-old man with nystagmus and tremor

   c. 42-year-old man with frequent polyregional attacks

   d. 40-year-old woman with MS since 28, with monoregional attacks with two pregnancies

37. All of the following suggest MS except:
    a. Gait disturbance
    b. Optic neuritis
    c. Negative Babinski reflex
    d. Presence of Lhermitte's sign

38. In a patient with MS you observe tremors, nystagmus, and ataxia. These symptoms are related to the:
    a. Optic nerve
    b. Brain stem
    c. Spinal cord
    d. Sensory pathways

39. In contrast to interferon therapy, glatiramer acetate:
    a. Has a higher incidence of laboratory abnormalities
    b. Is effective for secondary progressive MS
    c. Is not associated with flu-like symptoms
    d. Can result in long-term side effects

40. A rare but serious side effect of high-dose pulse steroid treatments is:
    a. Avascular necrosis
    b. Hypothyroidism
    c. Optic neuritis
    d. Tonic spasms

41. When assessing a patient who complains of cognitive difficulties, which of the following would you expect to see?
    a. Good long-term memory
    b. Intact general intelligence
    c. Good problem-solving skills
    d. Decreased short-term memory

42. In a woman age 32 who has had MS for 3 years, the risks of pregnancy can be explained as follows:
    a. Pregnancy will accelerate the course of your disease.
    b. You may experience an exacerbation during pregnancy.
    c. Pregnancy has no long-term effect on your disease course, but you may have an increased risk for a relapse in your early postpartum months.
    d. Your disease may become secondary progressive during pregnancy.

43. Why should people with MS be screened for depression?

    a. People with MS have a higher rate of suicide.

    b. Signs of depression can indicate an acceleration of the disease process.

    c. Depression can interfere with the effectiveness of medications.

    d. Depression is an unusual and serious sign in MS.

44. When assessing a patient with MS, which of the following is a primary symptom?

    a. Visual changes

    b. Urinary tract infection

    c. Skin breakdown

    d. Social isolation

45. Which intervention would be most effective to decrease the intensity of MS symptoms during the summer?

    a. Warm baths

    b. Aerobic exercise

    c. Well-balanced nutrition

    d. Use of an air conditioner

46. An outcome of spasticity management should include the following outcome:

    a. Improved coordination

    b. Decreased fatigue

    c. Increased strength

    d. Decreased clonus

47. Which of the following statements would indicate that the patient has bladder dysfunction?

    a. I void every 4 hours.

    b. I have difficulty getting up from a chair.

    c. I sleep through the night.

    d. I have to use a pad to catch my urine.

48. Which of these instructions would you give to a patient who is experiencing bowel dysfunction?

    a. The anticholinergic medication that you are taking will decrease constipation.

    b. Exercising your anal sphincter will give you bowel control.

    c. You should increase your intake of fluids and fiber.

    d. Diarrhea is common in MS.

49. In a patient experiencing fatigue, instructions should include:
    a. Increased fluids
    b. Avoidance of caffeine
    c. Regular rest periods
    d. Avoidance of exercise
50. When teaching a patient who has cognitive impairment due to MS, all of the following are appropriate except:
    a. Playing background music
    b. Using repetition
    c. Encouraging use of lists
    d. Teaching in a familiar setting

ANSWERS TO REVIEW QUESTIONS

1. c
2. d
3. b
4. b
5. c
6. d
7. c
8. b
9. c
10. b
11. b
12. d
13. d
14. d
15. c
16. b
17. c
18. c
19. d
20. a
21. b
22. d

23. a
24. c
25. b
26. b
27. b
28. b
29. a
30. b
31. d
32. c
33. d
34. c
35. a
36. d
37. c
38. b
39. c
40. a
41. d
42. c
43. a
44. a
45. d
46. a
47. d
48. c
49. c
50. a

C

Supplemental Readings and Resources in Multiple Sclerosis

Bennett, S. E., Bednarik, P., & Bobryk, S. C. (2015). *A practical guide to rehabilitation in multiple sclerosis.* Teaneck, NJ: Consortium of Multiple Sclerosis Centers and the France Foundation.

Ben Zacharia, A. B. (2011). Therapeutics for multiple sclerosis symptoms. *Mount Sinai Journal of Medicine, 78*(2), 176–191.

Birnbaud, G. (2009). *Multiple sclerosis: Clinician's guide to diagnosis and treatment.* New York, NY: Oxford University Press.

Bowling, A. C. (2006). *Complementary and alternative medicine and multiple sclerosis.* New York, NY: Demos Medical.

Bowling, A. C. (2014). *Optimal health with multiple sclerosis.* New York, NY: Demos Health.

Buckle, G. J., Halper, J., & Rintell, D. (2013). *Advances in multiple sclerosis primer.* Teaneck, NJ: Consortium of Multiple Sclerosis Centers and the France Foundation.

Burks, J. S., & Johnson, K. P. (Eds.). (2000). *Multiple sclerosis: Diagnosis, medical management, and rehabilitation.* New York, NY: Demos Medical.

Cassidy, C. A. (1999). Using the transtheoretical model to facilitate behavior change in patients with chronic illness. *Journal of the American Academy of Nurse Practitioners, 11*(7), 281–287.

Chitnis, T., Glanz, B., Jaffin, S., & Healty, B. (2009). Demographics of pediatric-onset multiple sclerosis in an MS center population from the northeastern United States. *Multiple Sclerosis, 15*(5), 627–631.

Consortium of Multiple Sclerosis Centers. *International Journal of MS Care.* Teaneck, NJ: Consortium of Multiple Sclerosis Centers. Retrieved from www.ijmsc.org

Cook, S. (Ed.). (2001). *Handbook of multiple sclerosis* (3rd ed.). New York, NY: Marcel Decker.

Costello, K., & Halper, J. (Eds). (2008). *Multiple sclerosis: Best practices in nursing care—Disease management, pharmacologic treatment, nursing research* (3rd ed.). New York, NY: Bioscience Communications.

Courts, N. J., Newton, A. N., & McNeal, L. J. (2005). Husbands and wives living with multiple sclerosis. *Journal of Neuroscience Nursing, 37*(1), 20–27.

Coyle, P. K., & Halper, J. (2001). *Meeting the challenge of progressive multiple sclerosis.* New York, NY: Demos Medical.

Coyle, P. K., & Halper, J. (2007). *Living with progressive multiple sclerosis.* New York, NY: Demos Medical.

Coyle, P. K., & Rizvi, S. (2011). *Multiple sclerosis and related disorders.* New York, NY: Springer Publishing Company.

Farrell, P. (2010). *It's not all in your head.* New York, NY: Demos Medical.

Files, D. K., Jausurawond, T., Katriajian, R., & Danoff, R. (2015). Multiple sclerosis. *Primary Care, 42*(2), 159–175.

Filippi, M., Rovaris, M., & Comi, G. (2007). *Neurodegeneration in multiple sclerosis.* New York, NY: Springer Publishing Company.

Fishman, L. (2007). *Yoga and multiple sclerosis.* New York, NY: Demos Medical.

Gingold, J. (2008). *Mental sharpening stones.* New York, NY: Demos Medical.

Goldberg, S. (1979). *Clinical neuroanatomy made ridiculously simple.* Miami, FL: Med Master.

Goldman Consensus Group. (2005). The Goldman Consensus statement on depression in multiple sclerosis. *Multiple Sclerosis, 11,* 328-332.

Halper, J. (Ed.). (2007). *Advanced concepts in multiple sclerosis nursing.* New York, NY: Demos Medical.

Halper, J., & Holland, N. J. (2011). *Comprehensive nursing care in multiple sclerosis* (3rd ed.). New York, NY: Demos Medical.

Holland, N. J., & Halper, J. (Eds.). (2005). *Multiple sclerosis: A self-care guide to wellness.* New York, NY: Demos Medical.

Holland, N. J., & Madonna, M. (2005). Nursing grand rounds: Multiple sclerosis. *Journal of Neuroscience Nursing, 37*(1), 15–19.

Holland, N. J., Murray, T. J., & Reingold, S. C. (2007). *Multiple sclerosis: A guide for the newly diagnosed.* New York, NY: Demos Medical.

Kalb, R. C. (Ed.). (2005). *Multiple sclerosis: A guide for families.* New York, NY: Demos Medical.

Kalb, R. C. (Ed.). (2007). *Multiple sclerosis: The questions you have—The answers you need.* New York, NY: Demos Medical.

LaRocca, N. (2006). *Multiple sclerosis: Understanding the cognitive challenges.* New York, NY: Demos Medical.

Lowenstein, N. (2009). *Fighting fatigue in multiple sclerosis.* New York, NY: Demos Medical.

Lublin, F. D., & Reingold, S. C. (1996). Defining the course of multiple sclerosis: Results of an international survey. *Neurology, 46,* 907–911.

Luccinetti, C. F., & Hohlfeld, R. (2010). *Multiple sclerosis 3: Blue books of neurology.* New York, NY: Saunders Elsevier.

Multiple Sclerosis Nurse Specialist Consensus Committee. (2008). *Best practices in nursing care: Disease management, pharmacological treatment, nursing research.* New York, NY: Bioscience.

Multiple Sclerosis Nurse Specialist Consensus Committee. (2010a). *Multiple sclerosis: Key issues in nursing management: Adherence, cognitive function, quality of life.* New York, NY: EME.

Multiple Sclerosis Nurse Specialist Consensus Committee. (2010b). *Advanced practice nursing in multiple sclerosis: Advanced skills, advancing responsibilities.* New York, NY: EME.

Murray, T. J. (2006). *Multiple sclerosis: The history of a disease.* New York, NY: Demos Medical.

National Institute of Medicine. (2001). *Multiple sclerosis: Current status and strategies for the future.* Washington, DC: Author.

Olek, M. (Ed.). (2005). *Multiple sclerosis: Etiology, diagnosis, and new treatment strategies.* New York, NY: Springer Publishing Company.

Paty, D., & Ebers G. C. (Eds.). (1998). *Multiple sclerosis.* Philadelphia, PA: F. A. Davis.

Perkins, L. (2008). *Multiple sclerosis: Your legal rights.* New York, NY: Demos Medical.

Petzold, A., de Boer, J. F., Schippling, S., Vermersch, P., Kardon, R., Green, A., . . . Polman, C. (2010). Optical coherence tomography in multiple sclerosis: A systematic review and meta-analysis. *Lancet Neurology, 9*(9), 921–932.

Polman, C. H., Reingold, S. C., Banwell, B., Clanet, M., Cohen, J. A., Filippi, M., . . . Wolinsky, J. S. (2011). Diagnostic criteria for multiple sclerosis: 2010 revisions to the McDonald criteria. *Annals of Neurology, 69*(2), 292–302.

Polman, C. H., Thompson, A. J., Murray, G. J., & McDonald, I. W. (2001). *Multiple sclerosis: The guide to treatment and management* (5th ed.). New York, NY: Demos Medical.

Rao, S. M., Leo, G. J., Bernardin, L., & Unverzagt, F. (1991). Cognitive dysfunction in multiple sclerosis: I: Frequency, patterns, and prediction. *Neurology, 41,* 685–691.

Rizvi, S. A., & Coyle, P. K. (Eds.). (2011). *Clinicial neuroimmunology: Multiple sclerosis and related disorders.* New York, NY: Humana Press.

Rodriguez, M., Kantarci, O. H., & Pirko, I. (Eds). (2013). *Multiple sclerosis.* New York, NY: Oxford University Press.

Rudick, R., & Goodkin, D. (Eds.) (1999). *Multiple sclerosis therapeutics.* London, UK: Martin Dunitz.

Rumrill, P. D. (2008). *Employment issues in multiple sclerosis.* New York, NY: Demos Medical.

Saunders, C. (2001). *What nurses know: Multiple sclerosis.* New York, NY: Demos Medical.

Schapiro, R. T. (2007). *Symptom management in multiple sclerosis.* New York, NY: Demos Medical.

Schwartz, S. (2006). *Multiple sclerosis: 300 tips for making life easier.* New York, NY: Demos Medical.

Sheehan, G., & Barnes, M. P. (Eds.). (1998). *Spasticity rehabilitation.* London, UK: Churchill Communications Europe.

Stachowiak, J. (2009). *The multiple sclerosis manifesto.* New York, NY: Demos Medical.

Thompson, A. J., Polman, C., & Hohlfeld, R. (Eds.). (1997). *Multiple sclerosis: Clinical challenges and controversies.* London, UK: Martin Dunitz.

Thompson, A. J., Toosy, A. T., & Cicarelli, O. (2010, December). Pharmacological management of symptoms in multiple sclerosis: Current approaches and future directions. *Lancet Neurology, 9*(12), 1182–1199.

Van den Noort, S., & Holland, N. J. (Eds.). (1999). *Multiple sclerosis in clinical practice.* New York, NY: Demos Medical.

Waubant, E. L. (Ed). (2011). *Multiple sclerosis.* New York, NY: Saunders Elsevier.

Weiner, H. (2004). *Curing MS.* New York, NY: Crown.

Whitaker-McFarlin, M. S., & The Colloquium. (2004). *Topics in multiple sclerosis: Immunology and MS.* Somerville, NJ: Embryon.

Whitaker-McFarlin, M. S., & The Colloquium. (2005). *Topics in multiple sclerosis: The role of magnetic resonance imaging in multiple sclerosis.* Somerville, NJ: Embryon.

Zorzon, M., Zivadinov, R., Bosco, A., Bragadin, L. M., Moretti, R., Bonfigli, L., et al. (1999). Sexual dysfunction in multiple sclerosis: A case-control study: I: Frequency and comparison of groups. *Multiple Sclerosis, 5*(6), 418–427.

CLINICAL PRACTICE GUIDELINES

Consortium for Spinal Cord Medicine. (1998). *Neurogenic bowel management in adults with spinal cord injury.* Washington, DC: Paralyzed Veterans of America.

Disease-modifying therapies in multiple sclerosis. (2001). Washington, DC: Paralyzed Veterans of America.

Fatigue in multiple sclerosis. (1999). Washington, DC: Paralyzed Veterans of America.

Immunizations in multiple sclerosis. (2001). Washington, DC: Paralyzed Veterans of America.

Multiple Sclerosis Council for Clinical Practice Guidelines. (2005). *Spasticity management in multiple sclerosis* (2nd ed.). Teaneck, NJ: Consortium of Multiple Sclerosis Centers.

Urinary dysfunction and multiple sclerosis. (1999). Washington, DC: Paralyzed Veterans of America.

WHITE PAPERS

Advocacy in multiple sclerosis. (2010). Consortium of Multiple Sclerosis Centers. Retrieved from www.mscare.org

Comprehensive care in multiple sclerosis. (2010). Consortium of Multiple Sclerosis Centers. Retrieved from www.mscare.org

Self-management in multiple sclerosis. (2010). Consortium of Multiple Sclerosis Centers. Retrieved from www.mscare.org

WEB RESOURCES

Accelerated Cure Project for MS
http://acceleratedcure.org
American Academy of Neurology
www.aan.com
Can Do Multiple Sclerosis
www.mscando.org
The Consortium of Multiple Sclerosis Centers
www.mscare.org
European Committee for Treatment and Research in Multiple Sclerosis
www.ectrims.eu
The International Organization of Multiple Sclerosis Nurses

www.iomsn.org
Multiple Sclerosis Association of America
www.mymsaa.org
Multiple Sclerosis Coalition
www.ms-coalition.org
Multiple Sclerosis Cure Fund
www.mscurefund.org
Multiple Sclerosis Foundation
http://msfocus.org
Multiple Sclerosis Views & News
www.msviews.org
National Multiple Sclerosis Society
www.nationalmssociety.org
North American Research Committee on Multiple Sclerosis
http://narcoms.org
United Spinal Association
www.unitedspinal.org

D

Consortium of Multiple Sclerosis Centers' Recommendations for Care of Those Affected by Multiple Sclerosis*

Multiple sclerosis (MS) is a lifelong neurologic disease with far-reaching and variable implications for patients, their families, and their social and vocational sphere of influence. The disease course remains uncertain for each patient, symptoms tend to wax and wane because of a variety of causes, and treatment concerns range from physical to social to emotional and back again. This dynamic pattern of need for and the necessity of appropriate care call for a philosophy of care that, to date, has not been well articulated or published. The standards for symptom management and disease-altering therapies have been promulgated during the past decade on the basis of both research and expert consensus. Therefore, the Consortium of Multiple Sclerosis Centers (CMSC) has determined that basic recommendations for care are required in MS.

BACKGROUND AND VISION OF CMSC

The CMSC is the largest organization of MS health professionals in North America. It was organized in 1986 under the auspices of seven neurologists. Since then, it has grown to more than 180 member centers in the United States, Canada, South America, and Europe.

The CMSC includes numerous individual members who are neurologists, nurses, psychologists, and rehabilitation professionals. It has members that include academic centers, community programs, VA medical centers, individual health care providers, students, corporate sponsors,

*Source: CMSC (2009). Reprinted with permission

and nonprofit partners such as the Latin American Committee on Treatment and Research in MS (LACTRIMS, the Latin American counterpart of the CMSC) and Rehabilitation in Multiple Sclerosis (RIMS; the European counterpart), providing comprehensive care in MS. Today, it continues to experience tremendous growth.

The vision of the CMSC is to be the preeminent organization of MS professionals. Through collaborative and interdisciplinary approaches, this group will lead the development and dissemination of scientifically based knowledge regarding MS clinical care. The ultimate goal is to improve the lives of those affected by MS.

To that end, the CMSC engages in activities that consist of professional education, clinical research, advocacy, and communication of activities to the health care community. CMSC is particularly interested in the future of chronic care and the role of alternative care in the 21st century. The CMSC/North American Research Committee on Multiple Sclerosis (NARCOMS) patient registry seeks to identify treatment trends and demographic characteristics of patients throughout the world.

The print and virtual journal of the CMSC, entitled *The International Journal of MS Care,* is the official publication of the CMSC, as well as that of RIMS. All CMSC members receive subscriptions as part of their membership. It is a peer-reviewed journal with opportunities for special issues, supplements, advertising, and both scientific and clinical articles.

REVIEW OF LITERATURE

The CMSC identified a need to provide a document that describes comprehensive care guidelines for those affected by MS. An extensive review of the literature was conducted and revealed that very little had been written in North America about the care for those affected by MS from a diagnostic continuum perspective. Most of the literature in North America is directed toward current disease-modifying agents.

In a joint publication by the Multiple Sclerosis Society of Great Britain and Northern Ireland and the MS Professional Network, an absence of continued care after the initial diagnosis of MS was identified. The document described the various phases of MS and associated recommendations for care, and the importance of proper care and support through the various stages of the illness.

Another UK document, written by the Neurologic Alliance, outlined standards of care for people living with a neurologic condition. Although the focus of this writing is not solely on MS, it acknowledges the existence of a need for coordinated, patient-centered services that ensure continuity of comprehensive care.

One final article written by the European Federation of Neurologic Societies and published in the European *Journal of Neurology* cited the inconsistency and nonexistence of care standards for those affected by MS across Europe. The document illustrated the minimum standards of care for MS. The authors conclude that a significant improvement in care and support can be recognized through the application of standards.

The current trend in the North American literature related to standards of care is directed toward the concept of evidence-based practice (EBP). The impetus for EBP comes from payor and health care facility pressures for cost containment, greater availability of information, and greater consumer savvy about treatment and care options.

Simply stated, EBP means "integrating the best available research evidence with information about patient preferences, clinician skill level, and available resources to make decisions about patient care" (Ciliska, Pinelli, DiCenso, & Cullum, 2001) A comprehensive definition of the EBP approach "incorporates hierarchical ratings of multiple forms of clinical evidence (e.g., randomized controlled trials, systematic reviews, and meta-analyses) that represent a body of data subjected to rigorous systematic analysis of study design and methodology to minimize bias and validate reported findings" (DeBourgh, 2001). From this body of evidence, clinical practice guidelines are generated to suggest clinical decisions and the prescription of interventions for specific clinical situations.

The literature provides research that correlates the use of EBP with improved clinical outcomes. This research centers on the clinical management of the patient using guidelines or standards of care. Two of the thousands of citations related to improved clinical outcomes can be found in the cardiac population and in pediatric pain management.

The Joint Commission on Accreditation of Healthcare Organizations (JCAHO) has revised the proposed standards for disease-specific care certification in the ambulatory environment. A delineation of the JCAHO expectations for patient care management includes the following:

> Disease management is an interdisciplinary, continuum-based approach to health care delivery that prevents or delays exacerbations or complications of an illness or condition. One of the ways that this is accomplished is by using a standardized method of delivering clinical care based on clinical guidelines or EBP. (Joint Commission on Accreditation of Healthcare Organizations, 2001)

Finally, the literature is abundant on issues that have a direct impact on patient safety outcomes. This has been brought to the forefront by reports done by the Leapfrog group and the Institute of Medicine's publication *To Err Is Human*. The literature supports EBP and its relationship to a positive impact on patient safety outcomes. Leape, Berwick, and Bates (2002) state that "there will never be complete evidence for everything that must be done in medicine. The prudent alternative is to make reasonable judgments based on the best available evidence combined with successful experiences in health care."

Based on several decades of clinical care, the leadership of the CMSC has addressed the needs of those affected by MS. This has been accomplished by the Clinical Care Committee through the promulgation and dissemination of the basic recommendations for MS care throughout the spectrum and lifetime of the disease.

PURPOSE

An extensive review of the literature, along with knowledge that is derived from education and experience, defined a critical need to recommend care for those affected by MS in North America. The emphasis of this care is on the concept of a *diagnostic continuum*. The model for this care is flexible and changes according to the needs of the patient. MS care is focused not on episodic management, but on care across the trajectory of the illness, which spans a lifetime.

The continuum begins when a patient presents to the health care system, and it is maintained throughout the patient's life. MS is not the definitive diagnosis in every case. The core of the model is the patient, family, and relationship sphere. The participation and involvement of the patient in this continuum of care are highlighted to promote adherence, empowerment, and self-actualization.

On behalf of the CMSC, the members of the Clinical Care Committee of the CMSC determined that the purposes of this document are as follows:

1. To provide a conceptual and practical framework for health care practitioners involved in the care of those affected by MS.
2. To emphasize the model of a diagnostic continuum of care in MS.
3. To present a format for this document that is "living," meaning that it will evolve and change over time as more research findings become available.
4. To motivate and direct research related to MS using the EBP framework.
5. To furnish supportive documents that broaden the scope of knowledge and understanding for the care providers of those affected by MS.
6. To promote adherence with JCAHO standards for disease management.

OVERVIEW OF MS

MS is a disease of the central nervous system. It has a far-reaching and variable impact on young adults and is one of the most common neurologic diseases of the younger generation. It strikes people in the prime of their lives, between the ages of 15 and 60 years. The highest incidence occurs between the ages of 30 and 50 years.

The hallmarks of MS are unpredictability, uncertainty, and loss of control. A variety of physical impairments can result in drastic changes in the patient's lifestyle, roles, income, productivity, family life, and emotional stability. Each person's prognosis is uncertain, and the course of the disease is unpredictable from one individual to another. MS has many symptoms and many related physical and emotional consequences that may affect function and quality of life. Lublin and Reingold have described the clinical course of MS according to four types based on clinical characteristics.

MS can have profound physical, social, and psychological consequences for patients and their families. It is a disease that has evolved from the mysterious "crippler of young adults" to one that has generated a great deal of public interest because of highly publicized treatments, both conventional and unconventional.

The impairments in MS are the result of demyelination in the brain, spinal cord, or both. These may be manifested in mild sensory symptoms, weakness, fatigue, bowel or bladder dysfunction, tremor, poor coordination, depression, and cognitive changes. These impairments can lead to limitations in a person's functional abilities (previously defined as disability and now as activity level in the World Health Organization terminology) and to restrictions in social, emotional, vocational, and sexual participation levels (previously referred to as handicaps). These disruptions can result from the disease itself or from inadequate health care and related services.

Health care in MS has grown and evolved during the past 20 years as knowledge and interest in this disorder have increased through advances in technology and the emergence of disease-modifying therapies. Before the mid-1970s, care was fragmented and provided in many locations. Patients received the diagnosis and medical treatment through a neurologist, treatment of bladder problems through a urologist, physical therapy and other rehabilitation care in another facility, and, less frequently, mental health services, neuropsychological, and vocational care somewhere else. The character of care at that time was "diagnose and adios." With the advent of MRI, that theme changed to "MRI and goodbye."

In the United States and Canada, until the early 1980s, few specialty MS programs or clinics were available. Little or no communication existed among health care providers, and minimal continuity of services was available. Patients whose mobility or lack of transportation precluded access to care received no ongoing care except for emergencies. MS care was fragmented, episodic, and related to crisis intervention instead of health maintenance. Treatment focused on symptomatic management, and disease modification was merely a dream. During the mid-1980s, with the advent of MRI, which facilitated the diagnosis of MS, and the approval of disease-modifying therapies during the past decade, care patterns have changed not only in North America but also throughout the world.

Comprehensive care in MS is an organized system of health care that is designed to address the medical, social, vocational, emotional, and educational needs of patients and their families. This care is provided by a team of professionals in one facility and tries to ensure that the direction and goals of treatment are consistent, logical, and progressive. The team approach facilitates a coordination of services and continuity of care, and avoids duplication and fragmentation for the patient and the family.

Comprehensive care embraces a philosophy of empowerment in which the person with MS takes an active role in planning and implementing health care and self-care activities and acts as consultant to the team. This active, rather than passive, role is fitting, in light of the fact that MS, like all chronic illnesses, is expected to last a lifetime. Persons with MS must learn to adapt and change in response to alterations in their physical functioning.

The comprehensive care team in MS consists of a well-informed person with MS, the family, relationship sphere, and care partners. The team may consist of a neurologist and other physicians, such as primary care physician, internists, urologists, gynecologists, orthopedists, ophthalmologists, physiatrists, as well as other professionals such as nurses, social workers, physical therapists, occupational therapists, speech-language pathologists, recreation therapists, psychologists, neuropsychologists, and clergy. This interdisciplinary team evaluates each patient individually and develops a plan of care that reflects individual function using the individual's input. This plan of care reaches beyond center or clinic walls into homes, workplaces, and places of recreation to enable full and independent functioning and a full quality of life. This vigorous plan of care reflects the ever-changing health care, social, and emotional needs expressed by the person with MS.

CMSC RECOMMENDATIONS FOR CARE

In the next two sections, a visual framework for care principles and principles of empowerment is presented. This is followed by the CMSC recommendations for care of those affected by MS for each phase of the disease that include:

- Clinical evaluation and diagnostic continuum
- Mild to moderate limitation in function
- Severe limitation in function

VISUAL FRAMEWORK OF CARE PRINCIPLES

The following graphic is provided to expand the visual framework of care principles for the reader. The model exemplifies the dynamics involved in the continuum of care required for those affected by MS. General principles of MS care provide the framework for care, no matter what the impairment or disability. Additional recommendations for care are based on the clinical status of the individual at any point in time. Because MS is unpredictable and impairment and disability can change because of the relapsing–remitting or progressive courses of the disease, the two-headed arrows illustrate the dynamic quality of the disease and its management.

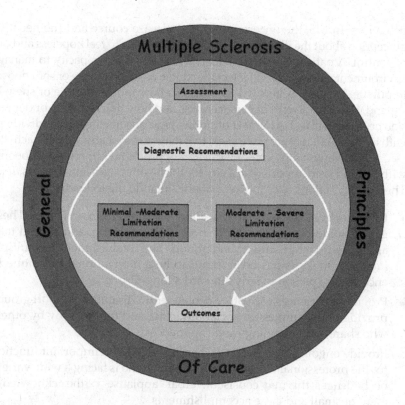

GENERAL EMPOWERMENT PRINCIPLES

The recommendations for care continue with information about the concept of general empowerment principles. These principles are critical to the care continuum. They should be used to guide assessment and treatment during any part of the disease process.

The word *empowerment* has been used frequently during the past decade to depict a wide variety of social movements, particularly those addressing the concerns of disenfranchised groups such as minority populations, those with disabilities, and women. The term *empower* is defined as "to give official authority or legal power and to promote the self-actualization or influence." In this case, *self-actualization* means maximization of the potential of those affected by MS.

MS is a chronic disease that changes an individual's life and self-perception. A person with MS, with the assistance of significant others and health care professionals, must manage symptoms, implement and adhere to or remain on prescribed treatments, and make modifications in lifestyle and behaviors to adapt to his or her illness.

It has been theorized that empowerment may be likened to the concept of self-efficacy, the belief that one can achieve desired outcomes through behaviors. In MS, the uncertainty of the disease course and the negative perception about the illness itself cause many people to feel hopeless and out of control. A patient's personal beliefs about his or her capacity to manage environmental demands will affect the course of action that he or she chooses to pursue. Personal beliefs will also impact how much effort he or she will expend, his or her length of perseverance, and how much anxiety or depression he or she will feel. A number of studies have documented that individuals with high self-efficacy are more likely to initiate and sustain a valuable activity.

Patient and family empowerment is of profound importance to people with MS and is an important activity for the health professional in this field. Therapeutic actions to empower patients include the following:

- Facilitate goal setting that will allow for mastery experiences. These goals should be realistic, both short- and long-term, and should take all relevant factors into consideration. The establishment of multiple incremental goals has been found to be a motivational technique to encourage a person to strive toward a long-term goal.

- Provide experiences with other people with a disability. Support groups provide opportunities for social modeling and for empathy by others who share similar feelings and experiences.

- Provide ongoing affirmation. "Cheerleading" is an important function for the professional working with a patient who is facing a wide variety of challenges; this may consist of verbal "applause" or the acknowledgment of small and large accomplishments.

- Maximize physical and psychological functioning. Optimal physical and psychological functioning are essential components in the enhancement of self-worth. A fatigued and depressed person is more susceptible to a sense of diminished self-worth and less apt to act on his or her own behalf.

- Provide motivation and encouragement that life has meaning. The MS professional's ability to provide a patient with encouragement and a positive outlook is an essential art of caring. "While presence and availability are crucial elements to encouragement, offering statements of faith can also be very beneficial" (Davidhizar, Bechtel, & Miller, 1998).

- Provide personal belief in the ability to cope. Genuine concern about one's patient is an important feature of MS care. A nonthreatening opening statement will invite your patient to share feelings and concerns. The MS professional can then elicit the patient's previous coping strategies and evaluate how effective they may be in the face of a chronic disease, activity limitation, or participation restriction.

Empowerment is essential for patients, families, and the health care provider when dealing with MS and its widespread implications. Self-efficacy, self-confidence, skill development, and effective communication are vital components and key features to promoting successful coping with this perplexing and vexing chronic neurologic disease. The trick to empowerment is to learn and to teach others to focus not on "what was" but on "what can be."

In support of the concept of empowerment, these principles should guide the care of those affected by MS. They are consistent and timeless. These should encompass the family and relationship sphere. Those affected by MS should have the following:

1. Full and timely access to health care
2. Timely and accurate diagnosis of MS, MS-related symptoms, and non–MS-related conditions
3. Accurate information and skilled advice provided by experts in MS care
4. Treatment that is timely, appropriate, and cost-effective
5. Continuity of care
6. Collaborative and interdisciplinary approach to care
7. Care that is sensitive to culture
8. Support for health-related quality-of-life issues (HRQoL)

Note: No consensus exists concerning the definition of *quality of life;* however, most agree that it is a multidimensional concept. HRQoL takes into account three important life domains: physical, psychological, and social functioning, and it considers a person's subjective perception of their well-being in these areas. Quality of life is normally measured by means of self-assessment questionnaires, some of which have been specifically developed for people with MS.

ASSESSMENT

It is critical for assessment to occur at each part of the continuum. Assessment should include the following key components:

■ Determine
  A. Current health status and HRQoL
  B. Care providers and home supports
  C. Patient's and family's physical, cognitive, emotional, and educational needs
  D. Financial, psychosocial, health care, and spiritual resources

■ Evaluate potential causes of symptoms
  A. MS-related
  B. Non–MS-related

■ Review care plan

A. Adherence to current treatment regime

B. Barriers to adherence and empowerment

C. Evaluate for rehabilitation needs based on the full range of functions and disturbance of those functions

D. Relationships with other care providers

CLINICAL EVALUATION AND DIAGNOSTIC CONTINUUM

The clinical evaluation and diagnostic continuum includes the prediagnostic, diagnostic, and postdiagnostic period. This waxes and wanes throughout the life cycle of MS and includes other diagnoses.

RECOMMENDATIONS

For patients who exhibit symptoms suggestive of MS:

1. Refer the patient to a neurologist, MS center, or MS clinic to establish and/or confirm the diagnosis of MS, according to diagnostic criteria (see Appendix C).

2. The results of the diagnostic evaluation should be communicated in an appropriate setting and in a timely manner.

Once the diagnosis of MS is confirmed:

1. Postdiagnostic contact should be maintained with the interdisciplinary team.

2. Information and support should be provided at an individualized pace.

    a. Offer supportive counseling options and informed advice.

    b. Discuss options for pharmacologic and nonpharmacologic management.

    c. Provide anticipatory guidance (genetics, family and career planning, etc.).

3. Use an interdisciplinary approach to establish a plan of care.

4. Promote wellness-focused activities.

5. Refer to local MS Society or local voluntary organizations.

MILD TO MODERATE LIMITATION IN FUNCTION

A mild to moderate limitation in the ability to perform normal activities may be transient (acute exacerbation), or permanent (incomplete recovery from relapse or progressive disease).

Recommendations

- Postdiagnostic contact should be maintained with the interdisciplinary team
- Information and support should be provided at an individualized pace
  A. Offer supportive counseling options and informed advice
  B. Discuss options for pharmacologic and nonpharmacologic management
  C. Provide anticipatory guidance (genetics, family and career planning, etc.)
- Modify plan of care
  A. Patients with acute relapses should have immediate access to appropriate therapy
  B. Access to appropriate disease-modifying therapies
  C. Access to current symptom treatments
  D. Ensure links with community resources (e.g., home care, social services, MS society)
  E. Ensure access to aids, equipment, transportation, and adaptations for home, work, and leisure
- Promote wellness-focused activities

SEVERE LIMITATION IN FUNCTION

Severe limitations in the ability to perform normal activities may be transient (acute exacerbation) or permanent (incomplete recovery from relapse or progressive disease).

Recommendations

- Postdiagnostic contact should be maintained with the interdisciplinary team
- Information and support should be provided at an individualized pace
  A. Offer supportive counseling options and informed advice
  B. Discuss options for pharmacologic and nonpharmacologic management
  C. Provide anticipatory guidance (genetics, family and career planning, etc.)
- Modify plan of care
  A. Patients with acute relapses should have immediate access to appropriate therapy

B. Access to appropriate disease-modifying therapies

C. Access to current symptom treatments

D. Prevent and, where necessary, alleviate complications (e.g., identify those at risk for skin breakdown, aspiration, nutritional compromise, sepsis [urosepsis], and cardiopulmonary complications [deep vein thrombosis, pulmonary emboli])

E. Minimize social isolation

F. Ensure links with community resources (i.e., home care, social services, and MS society)

   1. Access to aids, equipment, transportation, and adaptations for home, work, and leisure

   2. Access to personal home supports to maintain autonomy

   3. Access to respite, if required

   4. Access to age-appropriate long-term care facilities if required

G. Promote wellness-focused activities

OUTCOMES

The focus of this section has been on the recommendations for care of those affected by MS. Through the use of this approach to care and the management of care on a continuum, the following positive patient outcomes will be promoted and maintained. Those affected by MS will have the following:

1. A timely and accurate diagnosis
2. Knowledge necessary for disease management
3. Effective disease-management skills and strategies
4. Adherence to an integrated care plan that promotes empowerment
5. Functional abilities and safety measures maximized
6. Relationship with interdisciplinary team established and sustained
7. Optimal symptom management
8. Optimal HRQoL
9. Care management that stimulates research possibilities related to EBP

CONCLUSION

The ultimate goal of these recommendations is to improve the care, clinical outcomes, and quality of life for those affected by MS. This can be appreciated through timely access to care, accurate diagnosis, successful symptom and disease management, an interdisciplinary approach to the plan of care, maximized functional abilities, and attention to practices that promote safety. Regional differences and cultural diversity in the care of those affected by MS cannot be ignored. Additional benefits from these recommendations include increased education of health care providers and payers. It is anticipated that the deployment of this model will promote standardization and efficiency that will influence a reduction in health care costs.

This publication is presented as a living document. It will continue to develop and grow as more knowledge and experience are gained in the care of those affected by MS. Consequently, the opportunities to engage in research will be plentiful as the management of care improves. The cumulative effect of improved clinical management and research will drive EBP and the sustained improvement in patient outcomes.

REFERENCES

Ciliska, D., Pinelli, J., DiCenso, A., & Cullum, N. (2001). Resources to enhance evidence-based nursing practice, *American Association of Critical Care Nurses Clinical Issues, 12*(4), 520–527.

Davidhizar, R., Bechtel, G. A., & Miller, S. W. (1998). Promoting self-efficacy in the chronically disabled client. *The Journal of Care Management, 2*, 56–57.

DeBourgh, G. (Ed.). (2001). Evidence-based practice: Fad or functional paradigm? *American Association of Critical Care Nurses Clinical Issues, 12*(4), 463–467.

Joint Commission on Accreditation of Healthcare Organizations. (2001). Proposed standards for disease-specific care certification.

Leape, L., Berwick, D., & Bates, D. (2002). What practices will most improve safety? Evidence–based medicine meets patient safety. *JAMA, 288*(4), 507.

Lublin, F. D., & Reingold, S. C. (1996). Defining the clinical course of multiple sclerosis: Results of an international survey. *Neurology, 46*(2), 907–911.

E

Clinical Course of Multiple Sclerosis

CLINICAL COURSES OF MULTIPLE SCLEROSIS (MS)

Based on a publication in *Neurology 1996*

Relapsing–Remitting MS (85% of people begin with this course)

- Relapse defined as the appearance of new symptoms or a worsening of old symptoms, lasting at least 48 hours in the absence of fever, not associated with a withdrawal from steroids and preceded by stability for at least a month
- In relapsing–remitting MS, relapses occur with full or partial recovery and disease stability between attacks

Secondary Progressive MS (50% of people with relapsing–remitting MS will convert to secondary progressive MS over time)

- Begins with relapsing MS, but, after some time, no period of stability occurs
- May have relapses, but symptoms will progress or get worse between relapses

Primary Progressive MS (occurs in 15% of people with the disease)

- Symptoms of MS begin gradually and slowly worsen over time
- Some stable periods may occur

■ Often difficult to diagnose

■ Limited treatment options

Progressive Relapsing MS (occurs in 5% of people with the disease)

■ Primary progressive onset followed by one or more relapses later in disease.

Reproduced with permission from Lublin, F. D., & Reingold, S. C. (1996). Defining the clinical course of multiple sclerosis: Results of an international survey. *Neurology, 46*(2), 907–911.

CLINICAL COURSES OF MS REVISED 2013

New Disease Courses—Clinically Isolated Syndrome

■ Not included in initial MS clinical descriptors

■ Now recognized as the first clinical presentation

   ● Characteristics of inflammatory demyelination

   ● Has yet to fulfill criteria of dissemination in time

   ● Shown to carry high risk for meeting diagnostic criteria for MS

   ● Use of the 2010 revisions to the McDonald MS diagnostic criteria may facilitate diagnosis using dissemination in time and space

   ● 2013 disease modifier phenotypes—active and/or not active

      ● Use of MRI

      ● Patient self-report +/−

      ● Expanded Disability Status Scale (EDSS)

■ Radiologically isolated syndrome

   ● More complicated where incidental imaging findings suggest inflammatory demyelination in the absence of clinical signs or symptoms

   ● May raise suspicion of MS

   ● Patients should be followed prospectively

   ● Should not be considered a distinct MS phenotype

Redefining Current Disease Classifications

■ Relapsing remitting disease (RRMS)

   ● Either active or not active

- Activity determined by clinical relapses and/or MRI activity (contrast-enhancing lesions; new or equivocally enlarging T2 lesions assessed at least annually)
- If assessments are not available, activity is "indeterminate"
- Progressive disease
  - Primary progressive—progressive accumulation of disability from onset (PP)
    - Active and with progression
    - Active but without progression
    - Not active but with progression
    - Not active and without progression (stable disease)
  - Secondary progressive—progressive accumulation of disability after initial relapsing course
    - Active and with progression
    - Active but without progression
    - Not active but with progression
    - Not active and without progression (stable disease)
  - Activity determined by clinical relapses assessed at least annually
  - MRI activity (contrast-enhancing lesions)
  - New and unequivocally enlarging T2 lesions
  - Progression measured by clinical evaluation at least annually
  - If assessments are not available, activity and progression are "indeterminate"

- The prior category of Progressive Relapsing MS can be eliminated since subjects so categorized would now be classified as PP MS with disease activity.
- The terms "benign" and "malignant" disease should be used with caution.
- Further research is needed to better define the value of imaging and biological markers in assessing, confirming, or revising MS descriptions.

Republished with permission of Wolters Kluwer, Inc., from Defining the clinical course of multiple sclerosis: Results of an international survey, Lublin, F. D., & Reingold, S. C. Neurology, 46(2), 907-911 © 1996; permission conveyed through Copyright Clearance Center, Inc. Reproduced with permission of American Acadamy of Neurology in the format Book via Copyright Clearance Center.

F

Multiple Sclerosis Diagnostic Criteria: An Evolution

SCHUMACHER 1965

- Clinically definite, probable, possible multiple scelrosis (MS)
  A. Based on age (10–50 years)
  B. Objective neurologic signs on examination
  C. Neurologic symptoms and signs that are of central nervous system white matter origin
  D. Dissemination in time—two or more attacks lasting at least 24 hours and separated by at least 1 month or progression of signs and symptoms over 6 months
  E. Dissemination in space
  F. No other explanation for symptoms

- Clinically definite if five of six criteria met—always including the last criterion

Reproduced with permission from Schumacher, G. A., Beebe, G., & Kibler, R. F. (1965). Problems of experimental trials of therapy in multiple sclerosis. *Annals of the New York Academy of Science, 122,* 552–568. John Wiley & Sons, Inc.

POSER 1983

- Another committee convened as new technological advances allowed the identification of lesions that were not clinically evident
- Allowed for "paraclinical" lesions: Those identified by evoked response testing or neuroimaging

■ Defined a laboratory-supported MS diagnosis

■ Based on positive cerebrospinal fluid (CSF) findings

A. Elevated immunoglobulin (IgG) levels, increased IgG index, presence of oligoclonal bands

Reproduced with permission from Poser, S., Paty, D. W., & Scheinburg, L. (1983). New diagnostic criteria for multiple sclerosis: Guidelines for research protocols. *Annals of Neurology, 13*, 227–231. John Wiley & Sons.

THE MCDONALD 2001 DIAGNOSTIC CRITERIA

■ Large international committee funded by the National Multiple Sclerosis Society (NMSS) and the International Federation of Multiple Sclerosis Societies (IFMSS) convened to revise diagnostic criteria to include new technology

■ Preserves traditional diagnostic criteria of two attacks of disease separated in space and time

■ Must be no better explanation

■ Adds specific MRI criteria, CSF findings, and analysis of evoked potentials as means of identifying the second "attack"

■ The group concluded that the outcome of the diagnostic workup should yield one of three outcomes:

A. MS

B. Possible MS (if not completely clear)

C. Not MS

MCDONALD MRI CRITERIA 2001

■ Abnormal MRI consistent with MS, defined as:

A. Must have at least three of the following:

1. One gadolinium (Gd)-enhancing lesion or nine hyperintense lesions if no Gd-enhancing lesion

2. One or more infratentorial lesions

3. One or more juxtacortical lesions

4. Three or more periventricular lesions

5. One cord lesion = one brain lesion

■ MRI evidence of dissemination in time

A. A Gd-enhancing lesion demonstrated in a scan done at least 3 months following onset of clinical attack at a site different from attack

B. In absence of Gd-enhancing lesions at the 3-month scan, follow-up scan after an additional 3 months showing Gd-lesion or new T2 lesion

C. Other paraclinical evidence

D. Abnormal CSF:

1. Oligoclonal IgG bands in CSF and not in serum

2. Or elevated IgG index

E. Abnormal evoked potentials

1. Delayed but well-preserved wave form

- Monosymptomatic presentation

A. One attack

B. One objective clinical lesion

- Primary progressive criteria

A. Positive CSF, *and*

B. Dissemination in space:

1. MRI evidence of nine or more T2 brain lesions

2. Or two or more spinal cord lesions

3. Or four to eight brain and one spinal cord lesion

4. Or positive visual evoked potential (VEP) with four to eight MRI lesions

5. Or positive VEP with less than four brain lesions + one cord lesion, *and*

C. Dissemination in time:

1. MRI

2. Or continued progression for 1 year

Reproduced with permission from McDonald, W. T., Compston, A., Edan, G. (2001). Recommended diagnostic criteria for multiple sclerosis: Guidelines from the international panel on the diagnosis of multiple sclerosis. *Annals of Neurology, 50* (1), 121–127. John Wiley & Sons.

MCDONALD CRITERIA SUMMARY

- Two or more attacks
- Two or more objective clinical lesions
- No other explanation
- New criteria use MRI, CSF, or evoked-potential testing when only one lesion is found and/or only one attack or when onset is insidious neurologic progression

APPENDIX E Summary of 2010 Revised McDonald Diagnostic MS Criteria

Clinical Attacks	MRI Changes	Additional Information Needed to Make the Diagnosis
2 or more	2 or more lesions on MRI or clinical evidence of one lesion with reasonable evidence of a prior attack	■ Clinical evidence may be adequate but additional changes must be consistent with MS
2 or more	Objective clinical evidence of one lesion	Dissemination in space ■ One or more T2 lesions in typical MS locations in the central nervous system (CNS; periventricular, juxtacortical, infratentorial, spinal cord) Await further clinical attack(s) in a different area of the CNS
1	Objective clinical evidence of two or more lesions	Dissemination in time ■ Simultaneous, asymptomatic gadolinium-enhancing or nonenhancing lesions ■ A new T2 and/or gadolinium-enhancing lesion Await a second clinical attack
1	Objective clinical evidence of one lesion	Dissemination in space ■ One or more T2 lesions in at least two typical CNS locations
		Await further clinical attacks
		Dissemination in time ■ Simultaneous asymptomatic gadolinium-enhancing or nonenhancing lesion at any time ■ A new T2 or gadolinium-enhancing lesion(s) on follow-up MRI (no timing required)
		A second clinical attack

0 progression from onset		One year of disease progression (retrospective or prospective and at least two out of three criteria)
		▪ Dissemination in space in the brain based on one or more T2 lesions in areas typical of MS
		▪ Dissemination in space in spinal cord based on two or more T2 lesions
		▪ Positive CSF

CNS, central nervous system; CSF, cerebrospinal fluid; MS, multiple sclerosis.

Source: Polman, C., Reingold, S. C., Banwell, B., Clanet, M., Cohen, J. A., Filippi, M., . . . Wolinsky, J. S. (2011). Diagnostic criteria for multiple sclerosis: 2010 revisions to the McDonald criteria. *Annals of Neurology, 69,* 292–302.

Index

Printed in the United States
By Bookmasters

Printed in the United States
By Bookmasters